The New Allergy Diet

The New Allergy Diet

The step-by-step guide to overcoming food intolerance

Dr J.O. Hunter

With Elizabeth Workman
and Jenny Woolner

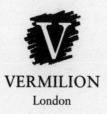

VERMILION
London

3 5 7 9 10 8 6 4

First, second & third editions text © Dr John Hunter,
Dr Virginia Alun Jones and Elizabeth Workman 1984, 1988, 1996
This fourth edition text © Dr John Hunter, Elizabeth Workman
and Jenny Woolner 2000

First published in the United Kingdom in 1984 by Martin Dunitz Ltd
Second edition published in 1988 by Macdonald Optima
Third edition published in 1996 by Vermilion
This fourth revised edition published in 2000
by Vermilion an imprint of Ebury Press
Random House, 20 Vauxhall Bridge Road, London SW1V 2SA

Random House Australia (Pty) Limited
20 Alfred Street, Milsons Point, Sydney,
New South Wales 2061, Australia

Random House New Zealand Limited
18 Poland Road, Glenfield, Auckland 10, New Zealand

Random House South Africa (Pty) Limited
Endulini, 5A Jubilee Road, Parktown 2193, South Africa

The Random House Group Limited Reg. No. 954009

www.randomhouse.co.uk

A CIP catalogue record for this book is available from the British
Library.

ISBN 0 09 182074 X

Papers used by Vermilion are natural, recyclable products made from
wood grown in sustainable forests.

Printed and bound by Mackays of Chatham plc, Chatham, Kent

About the authors

John Hunter is a Consultant Physician at Addenbrooke's Hospital, Cambridge and a recognized authority on the subject of food allergy and intolerance. He developed an interest in food in relation to diseases of the gut as a result of the need of the many sufferers of irritable bowel syndrome attending his outpatients' clinic. He has contributed over a hundred research papers to major medical journals including *The Lancet*, *Nature* and the *British Medical Journal*.

Elizabeth Workman gained her State Registration as a dietitian after following the dietetics course at Leeds Metropolitan University, already being a holder of a biological sciences degree from Leicester University. She has gained great expertise in helping people with food-related diseases and enjoys the challenge of devising appetizing and nutritious recipes from unusual ingredients, not least being because her husband is a vegetarian and she caters for a growing family. She is currently working in Cheshire as a community dietitian.

Jenny Woolner graduated from Southampton University with a degree in Biochemistry and Physiology with nutrition, and obtained her State Registration as a dietitian and an MSC in Health Sciences from Leeds Metropolitan University. She has worked as a research dietitian with Dr Hunter for the past seven years, contributing to a number of research papers, and currently combines this with bringing up her young family.

Acknowledgements

The authors wish to thank Mrs Pamela Harris for her invaluable help in designing the recipes.

Contents

Introduction

Food allergy is a term that the medical profession is wary of, and rightly so. A great deal of press coverage has led to the popular idea that any number of foods from avocado pear to zucchini can cause a whole range of 'allergic' reactions including rashes, runny noses and headaches. This has meant that people have been diagnosing all sorts of food allergies for themselves and may be in danger of nutritional deficiencies by excluding too many foods from their diets.

In this book we show how a number of conditions are known to be caused by intolerance to particular foods. We and other researchers have proved by medical trials that this food intolerance can be treated by putting people on to a diet excluding the ingredients that cause their symptoms. The diets need careful balancing to ensure that they are properly nutritious and healthy, and from our menu plans and recipes you will see that they can also be made appetizing and attractive.

Unfortunately, the foods that cause the conditions vary from person to person and discovering the true culprits can be time-consuming and difficult. Few doctors at present have experience in this field, so we have written this book to help people with various symptoms – and their doctors – establish whether or not they do have a food intolerance and, if so, how to deal with it.

What are allergies?

Most of the books written about food and disease call the condition 'food allergy'. Originally the word allergy meant an unpleasant reaction to any foreign substance in the body, but over the years it has changed, and now doctors use it to describe a reaction caused by a breakdown of the immune system.

The real job of the immune system is to recognize and destroy infecting agents such as bacteria and viruses that have got into the body. Substances in the blood called antibodies are produced and these make the cells defending the body attack the germs. In allergic reactions an abnormal type of antibody is produced that reacts to certain foreign substances called allergens, such as spores, pollens and foods. The combination of these antibodies with the allergen produces the allergic symptoms.

In most allergies doctors can detect the allergic reaction going on in the blood, but in the case of food allergy this type of reaction is hardly ever found. This is why doctors have doubted the existence of such a condition as food allergy. Yet some foods have been proved to cause diseases.

How do foods cause diseases?

In some cases the role food plays in causing disease is well established. For example, coeliac disease is a condition in which gluten, a protein found in wheat, rye and barley, damages the lining of the small intestine so that food is not properly absorbed. This leads to a number of difficulties including diarrhoea, bone disease and failure to grow, or loss of weight. Anaemia may also result from these problems. Because the symptoms can be caused by several other conditions it is not safe to start a gluten-free diet as treatment without being diagnosed first by a specialist.

Coeliac disease is thought to affect about one in three hundred to one in two thousand people in the UK. The discovery that coeliac disease was caused by gluten was purely accidental. Most of the wheat grown in Holland during the Second World War was directed to the German army at the Front, so the civilian population had to make do with potatoes. At this time children with coeliac disease made dramatic improvements, and the Dutch specialist Dr W.K. Dicke made the connection that excluding gluten from the diet had made the children better.

People with coeliac disease recover completely once they avoid foods containing gluten. However, they should still be seen regularly by their specialist to make sure they are well and not lapsing on the diet, even by mistake.

Commercial gluten-free products are available, but these are useful only to people with coeliac disease. Many of the recipes in this book are suitable for coeliacs and further help may be obtained from the National Coeliac Society.

Another condition in which there is a link between food and symptoms is lactose intolerance. Lactose is a sugar contained in milk which is digested by a natural chemical called an enzyme, found in the wall of the intestine. All children have this enzyme. It normally disappears in early adult life in African, Black American and Asian populations, and occasionally in Europeans. This means that some people may develop diarrhoea if they drink milk, because they are unable to break down the lactose.

Other foods contain chemicals that can upset some people. This may be linked to the way the various enzymes in their bodies behave. A clue in the discovery was the action of one of the enzymes called mono-amine oxidase. Certain drugs reduce its activity, and people who are taking them have to avoid eating foods such as cheese, red wine, yeast or yeast extract, otherwise they get high blood pressure and severe headaches.

Unfortunately, it is not as simple as that; food intolerance is not always the result of the behaviour of enzymes. There are other chemicals that work in different ways, including caffeine, histamine and tyramine. Caffeine is found in tea, coffee, cocoa, cola drinks and chocolate; histamine in cheese, beer, sausages and some canned foods; and tyramine in brewer's yeast, red wine and cheese. Too much strong coffee produces many familiar symptoms: restlessness, palpitations and heartburn. Histamine and tyramine may be a cause of migraine. It is thought that when they are absorbed into the body they may change the diameter of small blood vessels, and so bring on an attack in people who get migraine.

In our research in Cambridge we have studied food intolerance in the irritable bowel syndrome in great detail. People often develop IBS (see below) after a bout of gastroenteritis, or repeated courses of antibiotics. Indeed, a recent study showed that as many as one-third of patients developing gastroenteritis went on to suffer long-term symptoms of IBS. In our experience, many patients with this condition demonstrate changes in the bacteria living in their intestines. It seems possible that these bacteria are responsible for the breakdown of food chemicals which cause IBS.

We tested this theory by studying the excretion of hydrogen and methane in patients with IBS. These chemicals can be produced in the human body only by the action of bowel bacteria. We found that, compared to healthy people, IBS patients produced large volumes of hydrogen and little or no methane. When we put them on the exclusion diet (discussed later in this book), this excess gas production fell to normal and symptoms cleared. Thus food intolerance in many cases of IBS is caused not by any allergy, but by abnormal fermentation in the large intestine.

As there are so many different causes of reactions to food, and as most of them are nothing to do with allergy, you will see why we prefer to speak of 'food intolerance' rather than 'food allergy'.

Conditions caused by food intolerance

As we have explained, from the present state of knowledge about how foods cause disease, it cannot be said that food intolerance is the cause in every case – there certainly are other known causes for all these conditions – but we and other researchers have shown by the success of our dietary treatment that food intolerance is one of the most common. If you or your child are diagnosed as having one of the conditions below, a special diet may be the remedy. But you must discuss this with your doctor, and if necessary your specialist, before you start excluding foods from your daily intake.

The conditions listed below are the ones that may be caused by food intolerance and are therefore potentially treatable by diet. These are discussed in more detail in the next pages and suggestions are given as to appropriate diets to try.

irritable bowel syndrome	rhinitis
migraine	cow's milk sensitive
asthma	enteropathy
eczema	some types of arthritis
urticaria	hyperactivity in children

Recently in Cambridge we have also been very successful in treating Crohn's disease (an inflammation of the intestine) through diet, but as this disease can be severe, any changes in diet should be made only under close medical supervision at a hospital specializing in the condition.

Irritable bowel syndrome

Irritable bowel syndrome is a very common condition which affects twice as many women as men; nearly one person in three in the UK suffers from it to a greater or lesser extent at one time or another. The symptoms are bad abdominal pain and distension, together with diarrhoea or a very variable bowel habit. As we said earlier, people often develop symptoms after a bout of gastroenteritis or taking long courses of antibiotics. Yet the various X-rays and blood tests are always normal, and this has led many doctors to believe that the condition has psychological origins. People who have had abdominal pain for many years without relief tend to find life very stressful, but seeing a psychiatrist does not usually stop the symptoms, and our experience in Cambridge is that over half of our patients suffering from irritable bowel syndrome have food intolerance. Of the first 182 patients we treated by diet, we were able to relieve symptoms completely in 122. We wrote to eighty patients two years later to ask them how they were getting on. Seventy-one replied; fifty-nine were feeling well on their diet, and six were still well and had gone back to normal eating. So we have found treatment by diet to be far the best way of calming the irritable bowel.

Although not all cases are caused by food intolerance – menstrual changes, too much or not enough fibre in the diet or short-term stress can bring on the symptoms – we believe that anyone with irritable bowel syndrome should at least try an exclusion diet.

For more about IBS and diet, see the following chapter.

Asthma and rhinitis

Asthma is a very common disorder, especially in developed countries such as the United Kingdom. The main symptoms are wheezing and difficulty in breathing, which may be accompanied by coughing. There are many causes of asthma, probably the most common being the house-dust mite. However, food has also been shown to be an important trigger for an asthma attack. In one trial it was found that food provoked asthma attacks in nearly 30 per cent of sufferers. Studies have shown that a wide range of foods can cause problems, with milk, eggs, artificial food additives and preservatives and wheat being the most commonly implicated. As asthma attacks can be serious, asthmatics, in particular children, should embark on an exclusion diet only under medical supervision.

Rhinitis is a non-infectious disorder where the sufferer has a persistently runny and stuffy nose. Like asthma, rhinitis has often been found to be related to food. In one study of patients with rhinitis, two-thirds were shown to be affected by food. In 19 per cent of these cases food was found to be the sole cause of rhinitis. In some patients the rhinitis was caused by various inhaled allergens with foods also having an effect. If your doctor is in agreement, it is certainly worth trying an exclusion diet (see page 42).

Migraine

Migraine is a very common problem. It is estimated that over five million people in England alone suffer from this illness. At least 90 per cent of people with migraine have attacks before the age of forty; most have their first attack during their teens or early twenties. In women there is a strong hereditary tendency and often a connection with the menstrual cycle. In some people the attacks develop quickly and last a few hours. In others they may be more drawn out, lasting one to three days. The headache is not always the main symptom of migraine and for many people nausea and vomiting are the major problems. Others also experience disturbed vision and flashing lights.

There are many triggers that can provoke or aggravate a migraine attack. Tiredness, stress, depression, shock, loud noises, bright lights and diet have all been implicated.

It is not only the types of foods we eat in our diet that are important, but also the frequency of our meals. Long gaps between meals can trigger a migraine due to the lowering of the blood sugar level. It is therefore important to have regular meals and snacks, particularly before strenuous exercise, such as bread, pasta, rice and potatoes, and proteins such as meat, fish, cheese, eggs and pulses. Sugary foods – for example, sweets and chocolates – provide only temporary relief, as they cause a rapid rise, followed by a rapid fall in blood sugar levels.

For hundreds of years migraine sufferers have also suspected that specific foods can trigger an attack. Some of the most common foods found to do this are cheese and dairy foods, red wine, yeast and yeast extract, chocolate and fried and fatty foods. These foods contain amines such as tyramine which, when they are absorbed into the body, may change the diameter of small blood vessels. This can bring on an attack in people who get migraine. The amines are also absorbed more easily when fat is present. This explains why fried food, dairy products, cheese and chocolate are often suspected of causing migraine attacks. Other foods such as tea, coffee and citrus fruits have also been implicated.

A study carried out by Professor Soothill at Great Ormond Street Children's Hospital in London showed a dramatic reduction in frequency of migraine attacks in children following an exclusion diet. He also found that these children had a problem with only a small number of foods.

Therefore, for migraine sufferers we recommend that an exclusion diet should be tried (see page 42).

Eczema

Eczema, also known as atopic dermatitis, is an itching red rash often found on the inside of the elbow and knee. The rash tends to come and go, and may scale over and form a crust. It is often treated with steroid creams and antihistamine pills. Eczema is particularly common in young infants and children, who frequently also suffer from asthma or rhinitis.

Studies have indicated that eczema can be caused by food

intolerance, possibly of an allergic nature. In children, the more severe the eczema, the more likely it is that food hyper-sensitivity is playing a role. Approximately a third of children with mild to moderate eczema are found to have food hyper-sensitivity. The most common foods involved are eggs and milk, but peanuts, soya, wheat and fish may also contribute to symptoms. In children with severe eczema 60 per cent are found to react to one or more of these foods. However, 85 per cent of young infants with eczema outgrow their food sensi-tivity by their third birthday. With your doctor's agreement a milk- and egg-free diet may be a sensible first approach. This must be closely supervised by a state-registered dietitian.

In adults, food sensitivity appears to be less common, with other factors such as house-dust mites, pollen, animal fur and moulds playing a more important role.

Urticaria

Urticaria (or hives) is a common condition in which large itchy red blotches (wheals) appear anywhere on the skin. In some cases sufferers may also develop angioedema or swelling, particularly of the lips and mouth. Very occasionally, this can be life-threatening if the throat becomes inflamed. These symptoms can last for as little as one to two hours or they may persist for many months, as in chronic urticaria.

Urticaria can occur at any age and in both sexes, but chronic urticaria is more common in adult women. The condition is usually treated with antihistamines. A number of factors can bring on urticaria, such as heat, pressure, water, cold, sunlight and physical exercise. However, in many cases foods, food additives and salicylates (a chemical found in aspirin and naturally in some foods) are known to provoke an attack. Although a wide variety of foods has been shown to cause problems, the most common are cow's milk, fish, eggs, cheese, yeast, chocolate and caffeine.

Therefore, we recommend that those suffering from urticaria should begin by trying a diet free from artificial colourings, preservatives and salicylates (see page 21).

If there is no improvement in the condition after one month, an exclusion diet should be tried (see page 42).

Cow's milk sensitive enteropathy

This mainly affects babies who are bottle-fed before the age of four months. The symptoms are the severe stomach pain known as colic, diarrhoea, eczema, vomiting and a runny nose. Babies usually grow out of these once they are on a solid diet, at about the age of two.

Mothers who think their children are reacting to cow's milk should talk to their family doctor. Although a cow's milk-free diet may be suggested by a doctor or paediatrician, children should never be put on any abnormal diet without close medical supervision.

Hyperactivity

Many children behave badly and it has become almost fashionable to call a child hyperactive who is simply energetic and noisy. But there is a clear distinction between overactivity, which is due to excessive energy, and hyperactivity, a condition that needs special treatment.

Very few children suffer from hyperactivity. The majority who have the condition are boys aged between one and seven. They demonstrate a sustained increase in physical activity together with poor concentration, impulsive behaviour and temper tantrums. Associated with this condition may be poor eating and sleeping habits, abnormal thirst and learning and behavioural problems. Many also suffer from headaches, asthma, hay fever and catarrh.

The most famous findings about diet and hyperactivity were made by Dr Ben Feingold in the United States. His diet, based on the elimination of artificial colours and flavours, aspirin and natural salicylates found in some fruits and vegetables, helped 30 to 50 per cent of the children he was treating to improve. Hyperactivity is also linked to other factors such as chemicals (found in aerosols, disinfectants, perfume, etc.) and dust.

Many paediatricians working with hyperactive children have dismissed the Feingold diet and at present there seem to be as many arguments against treatment by diet as there are for it. However, a study at the Hospital for Sick Children in Great Ormond Street, London, reported success with dietary treatment carried out in children with this problem. Of the seventy-six children treated, twenty-one recovered, forty-one improved and only fourteen showed no improvement. These children were put on a much stricter diet than Dr Feingold's. Not only additives, but foods such as cow's milk, chocolate, wheat, oranges, cheese and eggs were shown to affect the children. Sugar, which had been blamed by many previous researchers, was found to affect very few of the children.

With a child known to be hyperactive it would seem reasonable to start on the exclusion diet (see page 42). This excludes all the relevant foods and, by reintroducing the foods as instructed, the solution may be found. When dealing with growing children it is, of course, especially important to make sure that sufficient food, minerals and vitamins are provided. For example, calcium supplements may be necessary if a suitable milk substitute is not used.

Please note that a child should undertake an exclusion diet only with the approval, and under the supervision, of a medical specialist. The final diet must always be checked by a trained dietitian.

Artifical colouring-, preservative- and salicylate-free diet

'E' numbers describe both natural and artificial colours and preservatives. It is not necessary to avoid all 'E' numbers.

Check the ingredients listed on all processed and convenience foods, i.e. tins, packets, jars, bottled and ready-to-eat meals, for the following additives:

Artificial colours

Azo dyes are chemicals containing nitrogen and used as colourings in food, drinks and cosmetics. They may aggravate your condition so it is important that you avoid the following additives:

E102	tartrazine	E128	red 2G
E104	quinoline yellow	E131	patent blue carmine
E107	yellow 2G	E132	indigo
E110	sunset yellow	E133	brilliant blue FCF
E122	carmoisine	E151	black PN
E123	amaranth	E154	brown FK
E124	ponceau 4R	E155	chocolate brown HT
E127	erythrosine	E180	pigment rubine

Some foods may be coloured with natural colourings which can be included in your diet, such as E101 (riboflavin) and E160(a) (alpha carotene).

Artificial preservatives

Benzoates and sulphates are two main groups of preservatives added to certain foods by manufacturers. It is important to exclude from your diet E210–E219 (benzoates) and E220–E227 (sulphates). Also exclude the antioxidants E320 BHA and E321 BHT.

Try to include as many fresh foods as possible in your diet.

Salicylates

Salicylates are found in medicines containing aspirin, salicylate or salicylic acid. Your pharmacist will advise you about any medicines you buy. They are also found naturally in certain foods.

Foods high in salicylates are:

Berries such as blackberries, blueberries and raspberries;
 apples, oranges, pineapple, plums and rhubarb; dried
 fruit and grapes
Tomatoes, gherkins and cucumbers
All nuts, especially peanuts and almonds
Tea, coffee, wine, sherry, beer and cider
Liquorice, Marmite, curry powder, herbs and spices,
 Worcestershire sauce, white vinegar

Foods for an artificial colouring-, preservative- and salicylate-free diet

It is important to **check all labels carefully**, because ingredients of manufactured foods are liable to change.

	Not allowed	*Allowed*
Breads and cereals	Brown or white bread	100 % wholemeal bread, oats, rye, corn, rice; breakfast cereals free from colours and preservatives, e.g. Shredded Wheat, Weetabix
Crispbread		Wheat and rye based
Pasta	Caution: some pastas contain colouring, check contents on packet	Spaghetti, macaroni, vermicelli, etc.
Cakes and biscuits	Commercially prepared varieties, including special cake mixes	Home-made varieties using permitted ingredients
Vegetables	Canned and commercially bottled; tomatoes, gherkins, cucumbers	Fresh, frozen, dried, domestically bottled

	Not allowed	Allowed
Fruit	Berries, apples, oranges, pineapple, plums, rhubarb, grapes, dried fruit Caution: check frozen fruit and fruit juices	Fresh, frozen and bottled
Milk	Flavoured milk	Fresh, long-life (UHT), sterilized, skimmed, dried milk powder
Cream	Artificial creams	Fresh
Yoghurt	Coloured or flavoured yoghurt	Natural yoghurt
Meat and fish	Cured and pre-cooked meats, smoked fish, meat and fish products	Fresh meat and fish
Beverages	Squashes, beer, cider, wine, tea, coffee, fruit juices (see above)	Water, fruit and herbal teas

Arthritis

Many people are confused about the meaning of the word arthritis. It means swelling of the joints and there are numerous forms of arthritis, which may be caused by diseases as different as damage to the nerves or bleeding into the joints. No diet can help all these conditions.

Osteoarthritis is probably the most common form of arthritis, especially among women. Believed to be caused by wear and tear of the joints, particularly in the hips and knees. This sort of arthritis will not be helped by diet, unless of course, weight reduction has been recommended by your doctor, to alleviate the pressure on the joints.

Gout is caused by sharp crystals of uric acid forming in the joints. The uric acid comes from the breakdown of chemicals known as purines. Although most doctors now treat gout with drugs, which block the formation of uric acid or increase its excretion in the urine, some still supplement these with a diet which avoids foods rich in purines. These are found in protein-rich foods, in particular offal (e.g. liver, kidneys), peas, beans, sardines, pilchards, anchovies, herrings and fish roes. Gout was therefore one of the original forms of arthritis to be treated by diet. Treating rheumatoid arthritis by diet is not so simple.

Rheumatoid arthritis is a disease of the connective tissues, particularly affecting the tissues around the joints. It causes inflammation and, eventually, stiffening of the joint concerned. This form of arthritis is more common among women than men and affects up to thirty-eight women per thousand of the population at some time in their lives.

This is the form that has caused the most interest and controversy as far as diet is concerned. Several different diets have been promoted by doctors and herbalists, but unfortunately none has proved to be entirely successful (see page 24 for some examples of these). The role of diet in arthritis is far from established. Although a number of doctors have reported they have a few patients with rheumatoid arthritis who have found that foods have definitely caused their problems, a large number do seem to improve for a short time only because of the placebo effect – if they think the treatment is doing them good, it will. However, we have been successful in relieving symptoms in a number of people with an exclusion diet especially adapted for arthritis (see page 26).

Psoriatic arthritis is a special type of arthritis that sometimes affects people with psoriasis. The arthritis affects the lining of the joints, causing swelling, pain and stiffness. It usually affects only a few joints in the body. We have found considerable success in treating this with the exclusion diet for arthritis (see page 26).

Food supplements for arthritis

There are many supplements recommended for arthritis sufferers. The two most common supplements are fish oils and evening primrose oil.

The fatty acids found in oily fish such as mackerel, herrings, sardines, salmon and trout are used by the body to make chemicals which are less inflammatory than those made from fats in a normal diet. In this way the fish oil has a mild anti-inflammatory effect which may make it possible for people to take fewer drugs. Cod liver oil has been taken by arthritis sufferers for years; many people mistakenly believing that it 'oils their joints' and, thus, makes them more mobile. Scientific studies have shown some benefit for people suffering from rheumatoid arthritis when used in a concentrated form. Unfortunately, cod liver oil capsules from a pharmacist may not be concentrated enough to produce the same benefits. Also, the supplements used must be taken over a long period of time, at least three to six months, to be effective. However, if you are taking a cod liver oil supplement, *do not* exceed the manufacturer's dose as you could actually do yourself more harm than good.

Evening primrose oil acts in a very similar way to fish oil to produce an anti-inflammatory effect. However, there seems to be no advantage in taking both oils at the same time.

Other supplements often recommended for arthritis include ginseng, royal jelly, cider vinegar, New Zealand green-lipped mussel extract, selenium, garlic, honey and various vitamin supplements. These have not been scientifically studied and it is difficult to say whether they have any benefit. Often they are expensive to buy and may have harmful side-effects if taken in larger doses for a long period of time.

Arthritis: testing by diet

As we mentioned earlier, many different diets have been claimed to relieve rheumatoid arthritis. They are often based on diets eaten in countries where arthritis is rare. Unfortunately, most of these have been found to be disappointing.

Dr Dong's diet was devised in the 1940s and is based on a typical diet from China, where arthritis is relatively unusual. It is rich in fish and excludes red meat, fruits, egg yolk, dairy produce, additives, spices and chocolate. Although many people have claimed that the diet has helped them, a controlled trial failed to reveal any differences between those who followed Dong and those who ate an ordinary diet.

We believe that this diet excludes too many foods to be followed happily for a long time, and it lacks the flexibility of the exclusion diet – there is no point in avoiding a food unless you are quite sure that eating it causes trouble.

Because Eskimos eat a lot of fish, and very few of them suffer from arthritis, it has been suggested that enriching the diet with the polyunsaturated fatty acids found in fish might help arthritis sufferers. However, a study reported in *The Lancet* showed that the benefit was limited. The treatment group had less morning stiffness and fewer tender joints after twelve weeks on this diet, but when they stopped it they appeared to deteriorate more quickly than the other group, who received the average American diet. Besides, the relief experienced during the diet was far from complete. In our view there is little point in following a restrictive diet if it does not give total benefit.

The acid-reducing diet is based on the idea that acids produced in the body during digestion cause arthritis. It is true that uric acid is formed in gout (see p 22) but there is little other evidence to back this theory. The acid-reducing diet differs from Dr Dong's in that it encourages dairy products and avoids fish, tea and coffee. Apart from this it is very similar and lacks scientific support.

We are confident that people with arthritis who wish to try a simple dietary approach will come to little harm if they follow the diet laid out in the table on page 26 for three weeks. If your symptons improve over this time, you can go on to the reintroduction and testing of foods. The order in which you should test foods is shown on page 27. Each food should be tested for four days. If your synptoms do not return after this time, you can assume the food is safe and go on to try another food.

Foods for the exclusion diet for arthritis

(Foods eaten should be fresh or frozen. Canned food and packet foods should be avoided if they contain food additives).

	Not allowed	Allowed
Meat	Red meats, (e.g. lamb, beef, pork), bacon, preserved meats, sausages	Chicken, rabbit, turkey
Fish	Smoked fish, shellfish	White fish
Vegetables	Onions, tomatoes	All other vegetables, potatoes, salad, pulses, beans, lentils, peas
Fruit	Citrus fruit (e.g. oranges, grapefruit)	All other fruit (e.g. apples, bananas, pears)*
Cereals	Wheat, rye, oats, barley, corn, rice, ground rice	Tapioca, sago, millet, buckwheat
Cooking oils	Corn oil, vegetable oil	Sunflower oil, safflower oil, soya oil, olive oil
Dairy products	Cow's milk, butter, most margarines, cow's milk yoghurt and cheese, eggs	Soya milk, milk-free margarine, goat's milk products (e.g. yoghurt and cheese)+, sheep's milk products
Beverages	Tea, coffee (beans, instant and decaffeinated), fruit squashes, orange juice, grapefruit juice, tomato juice, tap water (except for cooking), alcohol	Herbal teas, fresh fruit juices (e.g. apple, pineapple), mineral, distilled or de-ionized water

	Not allowed	Allowed
Miscellaneous	Sugar, chocolate, yeast, Marmite, yeast extract, nuts, coloured tooth-paste, preservatives	Salt, herbs, pepper, spices (in moderation), white toothpaste, bicarbonate of soda, cream of tartar

*Some fruits, especially overripe ones, contain small amounts of yeast, but the quantities rarely cause problems.

+A few people find that goat's milk upsets them, so we now recommend soya milk in preference to goat's milk. You may find that you have no trouble digesting goat's milk products, but be wary of it if you have any sort of milk intolerance.

Reintroducing foods

When following the exclusion diet for arthritis, reintroduce one new food every four days in this order:

1. Milk
2. Tea
3. Tap water
4. Lamb
5. Rice
6. Butter
7. Onions
8. Beef
9. Eggs
10. Yeast – take three brewer's yeast tablets or two teaspoons of baker's yeast in water
11. Rye – test rye crispbread first then, if yeast was negative, test rye bread
12. Coffee – test coffee beans and instant coffee
13. Pork
14. Wheat – test as wholemeal bread
15. Chocolate
16. Citrus fruit
17. Tomatoes

18. Cheese
19. Corn – test cornflour or corn on the cob
20. White wine
21. Shellfish
22. Sugar
23. Oats
24. Yoghurt
25. Nuts
26. Preservatives – e.g. fruit squashes, canned foods with food additives, sausages, smoked fish, saccharin, etc.

It is very important for anyone following the diet for rheumatoid arthritis not to stop any pills that have been prescribed until it is quite clear that the diet has relieved the symptoms. If you do stop them too early you may suffer considerable pain. Again, we emphasize that it is essential to obtain your doctor's agreement before starting a trial to discover whether your arthritis can be helped by diet.

Testing for food intolerance

The main difficulty in treating patients with food intolerance is that the foods concerned vary greatly from one patient to another. Nearly all patients with coeliac disease will improve on a gluten-free diet; however, one patient with IBS may be better if they avoid chocolate and peanuts, whereas another is affected by dairy products. This variation causes much confusion. In order to simplify the problem doctors have tried to find a reliable method of testing for food intolerance. We describe some of these techniques below; so far, all have proved disappointing.

Skin tests were developed by the classical allergists of the early twentieth century. An extract of a suspected food is injected into the skin, either by putting a small quantity on the skin and pricking through, or by injecting a small amount immediately beneath the skin (this is called an intradermal injection). If the test is positive, the site of the injection will swell up and be surrounded by an area of inflammation. As only one skin prick is necessary for each food, a whole battery of tests may be done at the same sitting.

This type of test may be very useful when someone suffers from a genuine food allergy, but it will not cause a reaction in anyone who is, for example, lacking the enzyme which breaks down milk sugar. Despite a negative skin test, such a person would still show symptoms after drinking milk. Many people with food-related conditions such as migraine, diarrhoea and hyperactivity may have a negative skin test result.

As most people don't know the mechanisms by which their food is upsetting them, and as skin tests of this sort are by and large only available in private clinics which are expensive, they are probably not the best tests to begin with.

The tongue test is a modification of the skin test. Here the food extract is placed under the tongue to see if it provokes a reaction. We have found it to be disappointing and unreliable.

The radioallergosorbent test (RAST) is a more sophisticated form of the skin test. Blood from people with genuine food allergy contains antibodies to the foods concerned and these can be detected in the laboratory through a complex analysis. Again, this test will be negative for people who do not have a true allergy but who do have a food intolerance caused by a different mechanism. It has the same limited use as skin tests.

The cytotoxic test. In this test a sample of blood from the donor is mixed with food extracts. A few minutes later changes in the blood cells are observed under a microscope. As only a small quantity of blood and a small quantity of food extract are needed, a whole series of tests may be done on a single specimen of blood, so that the donor may be given a detailed report on possible food intolerances.

In theory, this test is enormously attractive, but we have found that in practice it, too, is of little help to people with intolerances. Researchers have not yet confirmed that the blood cells of people with food intolerance react against food chemicals, although they may in people who have true allergies. Most independent scientific studies have shown this test to be unreliable, and we have certainly found this to be the case. Many people come to see us claiming that they are unable to eat foods because their blood cells have reacted to samples of the foods in a cytotoxic test, but when they actually eat them, nothing untoward happens. For example, we gave wheat to a patient who agreed to do a 'blind' test. Although she had been told that she had a wheat intolerance, she had no reaction at all when she was given wheat to eat without knowing.

The hair test. Many laboratories offer to diagnose your food intolerances by analysing the minerals in a specimen of your hair. Minerals such as mercury, cadmium and arsenic are deposited in your hair as it grows. It is thought that a deficiency of a mineral can explain why some people react to certain foods. The amount of minerals in your hair sometimes reflects the amount in your body at the time the hair was formed – but of course in the case of people with long hair, this may have been many months before.

The link between mineral changes and food intolerances remains to be proved, and even if you have a hair analysis done you will still have to confirm yourself that the suspected foods cause trouble when you actually eat them. We do not recommend this technique. The main application of mineral analysis on hair is to detect the arsenic levels in murder victims!

Blood mineral analysis. A number of minerals are detectable in the blood and mineral analysis is offered by a number of laboratories on the same principle as detecting minerals in the hair. In practice, the significance of the levels of the various chemicals is poorly understood. Zinc is known to be very important for forming various enzymes and chemicals, and yet the way it works is still largely a mystery to us. Certainly, many people who are shown to have low levels of zinc in their blood in these tests don't appear to benefit when extra zinc is provided in their diet.

Since many of the other minerals being investigated are understood even less well than zinc, we do not have much faith in this type of mineral analysis for detecting food intolerance.

We believe that the only reliable way to detect food intolerances is to follow a carefully chosen but restricted diet, and see if symptoms improve. If they do, subsequent food reintroductions will show clearly which items cause a recurrence of the original problem.

Irritable bowel syndrome and the exclusion diet

Some considerations before changing your diet

If your doctor has diagnosed irritable bowel syndrome, changing your diet may be the answer to your problems. However, before embarking on an exclusion diet it is worth considering simple changes to your diet and lifestyle that may have important implications on your well-being. For example:

Do you tend to skip meals and grab a snack when time permits?
Do you eat very quickly?
Are you drinking enough fluids?
Do you drink coffee or tea continually throughout the day?

It is important to treat your gut with respect. Developing a regular meal pattern will help your gut to establish its own routine. If meals are missed, the signals that regulate bowel movements become confused. A large meal on a stomach that has been starved most of the day may result in an exaggerated stimulus to the bowels, which in turn can lead to discomfort and diarrhoea. Try to spread your food intake more evenly throughout the day. If your stomach starts to feel uncomfortable, stop eating; save a dessert until later. Some people find four or five smaller meals and snacks easier to manage than two or three large ones.

Take your time when you eat. Eating very quickly and drinking fluids at the same time makes it more likely that you will swallow a lot of air, leading to bloating and flatulence. Rushing around after eating diverts the blood away from your gut which may disrupt digestion.

Try to have regular drinks, aiming for a minimum of eight cups or glasses a day. This is especially important if you suffer from constipation. Fibrous matter in the intestine absorbs water, making it swell. This produces a bulky stool, which helps stimulate the bowel to push contents through the system. If you are dehydrated, stools will be small and hard, making them difficult to expel. Try to include drinks such as water, fruit juice and squashes. Some people find that carbonated drinks cause distention and discomfort. Caffeine, found in coffee, tea and cola drinks, can act as a powerful stimulus to the gut and make it difficult to relax intestinal muscles. It also has a diuretic action which has a dehydrating effect on the body. Try cutting down your caffeine intake and replacing such beverages with decaffeinated alternatives or herbal and fruit teas.

Certain foods can irritate the stomach. These may include very spicy foods, acidic foods such as citrus fruit and vinegar, or raw vegetables such as cucumber, peppers and onion. Alcohol may act as an irritant, especially on an empty stomach. Fried or very rich foods are also common causes of indigestion and heartburn. Another important point to consider is whether you are eating too little or too much fibre and this is discussed in more detail a little later.

Be aware that there may be factors other than food that are having an effect on your digestive system. The most important of these is probably stress. The connection between mind and gut is very strong and during stressful periods the intestine may be over-stimulated, making it difficult to function normally. Are your symptoms worse during the week, improving at the weekend or when you go on holiday? This may suggest a link with stress or it may reflect differences in eating patterns or types of food eaten.

It is not uncommon for people to hyperventilate without being aware that they are doing so. During the day large volumes of air can be swallowed in this way, resulting in bloating and discomfort. A physiotherapist can advise you on exercises to help you to breathe normally again.

Some women find their pattern of symptoms is related to their menstrual cycle and thus changes in hormone levels are likely to be playing a significant role.

It may help to keep a diary of when and what you eat and drink alongside a record of your symptoms. Include details such as periods of increased stress and the stage of your menstrual cycle. This should help you determine whether there are any links between these factors and your symptoms.

Fibre – too much or not enough?

High-fibre diets

A high-fibre diet includes wholegrain breads and cereals, vegetables, pulses (beans, lentils and peas), fruit, nuts and seeds. Foods containing fibre are important contributors of vitamins and minerals that make up a balanced diet. In addition, fibre itself has an important role. As explained earlier, it acts by absorbing fluids from the gut which causes it to swell. This produces a soft, easily passed stool. Increased stool bulk also helps stimulate the bowel wall to contract and push the contents through.

Not surprisingly, constipation-predominant IBS is the most likely variant to respond to an increase in fibre. The Western diet has a tendency to be low in fibre, owing to easily available highly processed and convenience foods. Dietary fibre should be increased gradually by including one or two new high-fibre foods each week. Rather than simply adding bran to foods, try adding a variety of fruit, vegetable and cereal sources. This ensures a good mixture of soluble fibre (found in certain fruits and vegetables, pulses and oats) and insoluble fibre (found mainly in cereal products), each of which has different beneficial effects on bowel function. It is important that you increase fluid intake at the same time as increasing fibre.

A high-fibre diet tends to be the first-line treatment recommended for IBS. There is, however, no evidence to suggest that people with IBS consume less fibre than those without. Fibre does not necessarily help all symptoms of IBS. In fact, some people find that their IBS becomes worse when they eat a high-fibre diet, especially when the fibre is in the form of bran. This is because fibre can act as an irritant. It is fermented in the large bowel by bacteria which produce gas. If too much gas is produced, it can lead to bloating, flatulence and discomfort. Too much fibre may also aggravate diarrhoea, as it speeds up the passage of food through the gut. A high-fibre diet should be tried for about four weeks to see if it is helpful. If the constipation is not resolved or if the high-fibre diet is not well tolerated, alternative types of fibre may be useful. These are known as bulking agents and are discussed on page 36.

Low-fibre diets

If you suffer from diarrhoea, bloating and flatulence, you may find a reduction in dietary fibre helpful. A low-fibre diet (outlined on page 36) works by reducing fermentation in the large bowel.

The low-fibre diet should be followed for four weeks. If you do not notice an improvement in your symptoms or you feel worse after this time, you should return to your normal diet. If, however, you are feeling better, you should try to reintroduce some fibre back into your diet following the guidelines on page 37. You may find that you tolerate some types of fibre better than others and you will therefore need to reintroduce these separately to note the effect. Build up the fibre to a level that you can tolerate. If you are unable to reintroduce much fibre you may need a vitamin and mineral supplement to ensure your diet is balanced and this should be discussed with a dietitian.

Bulking agents

It may be necessary to take a bulking agent while on a low-fibre diet to prevent constipation from developing. This should be discussed with your doctor. Bulking agents are natural sources of fibre that cannot be broken down to any great extent by the bacteria in the gut. This means that they have the useful property of encouraging regular bowel movements but do not contribute to the production of gas. There are several varieties of these including Celevac (methylcellulose), Fybogel (Isphagula husk) and Normacol (Sterculia). If one variety does not appear to help it is worth trying an alternative. It is essential that extra fluids are taken with these preparations.

The low-fibre diet

Eat your normal amount of meat, fish, eggs, milk and dairy products, fats and oils. These do not contain any fibre. For cereal products, fruits and vegetables, follow the guidelines below.

	Not allowed	*Allowed*
Cereal products	Wholemeal, granary and brown bread, bran, wholemeal flour and foods made with these	White bread, white flour and foods made with these
	Wholemeal pasta, brown rice	White pasta, white rice

	Not allowed	Allowed
	Wholegrain breakfast cereals, e.g. Weetabix, All-Bran, porridge, muesli and any cereals with added nuts and dried fruit	Rice Krispies and Cornflakes
	Wholegrain biscuits, e.g. digestive, flapjacks and cereal bars; biscuits containing nuts and dried fruit	Biscuits made from white flour, e.g. Rich Tea, wafers
	Wholegrain crackers and crispbreads, Ryvita, oatcakes	Crispbreads and crackers made from white flour, e.g. cream crackers
Fruit	All dried fruit, berries and bananas	All other fruit, maximum 2 portions a day; avoid skins and seeds
Vegetables	All pulses, beans, chickpeas, lentils, peas, sweetcorn, Brussels sprouts	All other vegetables, maximum 2 portions a day in addition to potato; avoid skins, seeds and stalks
Miscellaneous	Nuts, seeds	Fruit and vegetable juices (not prune juice)

Reintroducing fibre

Week 1

Try eating the skins on fruit and vegetables, e.g. apples, pears, potatoes.

Week 2

Eat an extra piece of fruit a day, e.g. a banana (but not dried fruit), *or* an extra portion of vegetables (not pulses). Five portions a day of fruits and vegetables (not including potatoes) are recommended long-term for a healthy diet.

N.B. One glass of fruit juice counts as one portion of fruit.

Week 3
Try replacing white bread with wholemeal bread.

Week 4
Try a higher-fibre breakfast cereal, e.g. Weetabix, Shredded Wheat or Bran Flakes.

Week 5
If you are still symptom-free, you may like to try dried fruit or pulses.

Remember, these reintroductions give a gradual build-up of fibre in your diet. The aim is to identify a level of fibre that you can comfortably take.

You may find that you can eat high-fibre vegetables on days when you do not have wholemeal bread and high-fibre breakfast cereals, or vice versa. If this is the case, try varying the sources of your fibre intake on a daily basis to achieve a balanced diet.

The exclusion diet
– an introduction

If you have found previous suggestions unhelpful, now might be the time to consider whether a specific food or group of foods make your symptoms worse. An exclusion diet will help you find out whether you have any food intolerances. It can be difficult to pinpoint individual foods because the ones that are most likely to upset you are the ones that we tend to eat every day, sometimes at every meal. If your symptoms are similar from day to day this will provide few clues as to the offending foods. Also, a food may need to be eaten more than once before symptoms are experienced and reactions may not develop for several hours or even until the following day.

Although some foods are more likely to be responsible for food-related symptoms than others, the only way to decide which foods upset you is to test them individually. Excluding one food at a time may not be helpful if you have more than one food intolerance. For this reason a safe, simple diet containing none of the common problem foods needs to be followed for a two-week period. If at the end of this you feel there has been a definite improvement in your symptoms, reintroduce the foods one at a time. If, however, you feel there has been little or no change, you should stop the diet and return to your normal diet. The next section will guide you through the exclusion and reintroduction stages of the diet.

How the diet was developed

Altogether, 584 patients with IBS took part in studies we carried out to develop the exclusion diet. Between 1979 and 1982 we studied 182 patients, using a very restrictive few-foods diet followed by the gradual reintroduction and testing of foods. One hundred and twenty-two patients reported a relief of their symptoms on this diet. A list was drawn up of the foods that upset these patients (see page 40). From this list we developed a less restrictive exclusion diet that avoided all the foods to which 20 per cent or more of the patients had been intolerant. This list was modified slightly following two subsequent reviews of the diet to produce the diet we now recommend. Approximately 60 per cent of all the patients who took part in the studies and completed food testing found they were able to control their symptoms on this diet.

Review of foods tested by patients attending clinic, 1979–1982

Food	Percentage of patients affected	Food	Percentage of patients affected
Cereals		**Vegetables**	
wheat	60	onions	22
corn	44	potatoes	20
oats	34	cabbage	19
rye	30	sprouts	18
barley	24	peas	17
rice	15	carrots	15
		lettuce	15
Dairy Products		leeks	15
milk	44	broccoli	14
cheese	39	soya beans	13
eggs	26	spinach	13
butter	25	mushrooms	12
yoghurt	24	parsnips	12
		tomatoes	11
Fish		cauliflower	11
white fish	10	celery	11
shellfish	10	green beans	10
smoked fish	7	cucumber	10
		turnip/swede	10
Meat		marrow	8
beef	16	beetroot	8
pork	14	peppers	6
chicken	13		
lamb	11	**Miscellaneous**	
turkey	8	coffee	33
		tea	25
Fruit		nuts	22
citrus	24	chocolate	22
rhubarb	12	preservatives	20
apple	12	yeast	20
banana	11	sugar cane	13
pineapple	8	sugar beet	12
pear	8	alcohol	12
strawberries	8	saccharin	9
grapes	7	honey	2
melon	5		
avocado pear	5		
raspberries	4		

Getting started

Before starting the exclusion diet, discuss your symptoms with your doctor to make sure he or she thinks this approach is sensible. Check that your doctor agrees that you have one of the conditions that can be helped by diet: it may be that you have another problem which has similar symptoms but needs different treatment. You should also discuss with your doctor whether or not you should continue with any pills or medicines that you have been taking. In general it is better to take as few pills as possible while trying an exclusion diet, as many contain starches as fillers, and they may be part of the problem.

First, consider how long it will take you to complete the diet and when would be the best time to start. The basic diet takes just two weeks but if you improve you will need to begin the gradual reintroduction of foods into your diet. This may take two to three months, depending on how many foods cause problems. It may, for example, be better to delay starting until a holiday or a particularly busy social period is out of the way. Be prepared to make some sacrifices; in the early stages of the diet take-aways are generally not recommended and it can be very difficult to eat out at restaurants.

You will also need to think about how you can fit an exclusion diet around work. It is unlikely that staff canteens or sandwich shops will provide suitable meals and you will therefore have to take your own food to work. You may also need to allow a little more time for lunch instead of having a quick snack on the run.

Balancing the exclusion diet with family life is another consideration. Will your family eat the same meals as you or will it involve cooking separate meals? Following a diet can be time-consuming: you will have to plan each meal, and cooking is likely to take longer, because few convenience foods are suitable. However, the recipes at the back of this book have been designed to make cooking on the exclusion diet as quick and easy as possible.

If you are vegetarian you may need to spend a little more time planning what you are going to eat as several of the staple foods of a vegetarian diet, such as dairy products, eggs and nuts, are excluded. Eat a wide variety of the vegetarian foods that are allowed to ensure your diet remains balanced, including a good mixture of protein sources from soya products, pulses, cereals and seeds.

On the positive side, following the exclusion diet is the best way to find out whether food is at the root of your problems. If it is successful, you will have found a cure to your symptoms that does not involve any medication. You will also have an opportunity to take a fresh look at your diet and to experiment with new tastes. You may even find you lose a few pounds in weight in the process!

The exclusion diet

For the first two weeks of the exclusion diet, you should avoid all the foods in the 'Not allowed' column and replace them with those in the 'Allowed' column.

	Not allowed	Allowed
Meat	Beef, meat products, e.g. sausages, beefburgers, meat pies, pâtés	All other meat and poultry, e.g. chicken, turkey, lamb, pork (including ham and bacon), liver, kidney
Fish	Fish in batter, crumb or tinned in vegetable oil	All other fresh, smoked and tinned fish, shellfish
Vegetables	Potatoes, onion, sweetcorn, baked beans	Sweet potatoes, all other vegetables, including salad and pulses

	Not allowed	*Allowed*
Fruit	Citrus fruit, e.g. oranges, lemons, grapefruit	All other fruit, fresh, tinned and dried
Cereals	Wheat, oats, rye, corn, barley (see pages 181–185 for foods containing these)	Rice, rice cakes, ground rice, Rice Krispies, rice noodles, rice pasta, tapioca, sago, arrowroot
Cooking oils	Corn oil, vegetable oil (may contain corn oil), nut oils	Sunflower, soya, olive, rapeseed, safflower oils
Dairy products	Cow's, goat's and sheep's milk and products, butter, margarine, cream, cheese, yoghurt, ice-cream, eggs (see pages 181–182 for foods containing these)	Soya milk and products e.g. dairy-free margarine, tofu, soya yoghurt, soya cream and soya ice-cream, sorbet (non-citrus); check labels
Beverages	Tea, coffee (including decaffeinated) squashes and fizzy drinks, citrus fruit juice, alcohol, tap water	Herbal and fruit teas, Ribena, non-citrus fruit juices, e.g. apple, pineapple, tomato, mineral water
Miscellaneous	Yeast (see page 184 for foods containing this) salad cream and dressings, mustard, vinegar, tinned or packet sauces, chocolate, sweets, nuts	Salt, pepper, herbs, spices in moderation (see page 60 and recipe section for alternative gravies, sauces and dressings); sugar, honey, syrup, jam (non-citrus), carob, Kendal mint cake, seeds, (e.g. Sesame snaps, halva, tahini).

Following an exclusion diet

Here are a few points to help guide you through the diet :

1. For two weeks before starting, record all the symptoms you have had, and when, to help judge the value of the diet later on.

2. For the first two weeks of the exclusion diet keep strictly to the list of allowed foods on pages 42–43. Remember, it is essential to continue for two weeks; because all traces of offending foods eaten before the diet begins must disappear from the body before symptoms clear, improvement is rarely seen in the first week. Don't give up; if you take a day off you will have wasted all your previous efforts, and will have to start again from the beginning.

3. During the first fortnight it is wise to exclude any foods besides those listed on pages 42–43 that you suspect have upset you; later on you will test and assess them properly.

4. During the second week you should eat as wide a variety of the 'allowed' foods as possible. This will help you notice any unusual food intolerances.

5. Throughout the two weeks keep an accurate diary of everything you eat and drink, which symptoms you have and when. Use a small notebook and allow a spread of two pages for each day (see below).

6. If after two weeks your symptoms have not improved, it is unlikely that food intolerance is the cause of your problems. Go back to normal eating, and ask your doctor about trying a different treatment.

7. If your symptoms have resolved you should proceed to the next stage of the diet: food reintroduction (page 45). If your symptoms have partially improved it may be helpful to continue the diet for just one further week, using your food and symptom diary to help identify any further food intolerances. Start to test foods only if you feel there has been an obvious change in your symptoms; otherwise, return to your normal diet.

Example of a food and symptom diary

	Foods	Symptoms
Breakfast 8.00 am	Rice Krispies, soya milk, apple juice	8.30 am Diarrhoea
Mid-morning 11.00am	Banana, peppermint tea	12.15 pm Wind
Lunch 1.15 pm	Chicken drumsticks, rice salad, lettuce, tomato, cucumber, soya yoghurt	2.30 pm Headache started
Mid-afternoon 4.00 pm	Camomile tea, pear	
Supper 7.30 pm	Pork chops, sweet potatoes, peas, carrots, soya rice pudding, Ribena	8.45 pm Bloated stomach 9.15 pm Diarrhoea

Reintroducing foods

Hopefully, by now you are feeling delighted by the improvement that the diet has brought. It is now highly likely that your symptoms can be controlled by diet. However, to find out exactly which foods are responsible still requires very careful planning. Continue to keep your diary throughout the reintroduction phase. The list on pages 47–48 shows the order for reintroduction. Try to keep to the following rules for reintroducing foods:

• With irritable bowel syndrome, migraine, asthma and rhinitis, we recommend that you reintroduce one food every two days. For constipation-predominant irritable bowel syndrome it may be wise to extend this period to four days. In the cases of eczema and urticaria a longer period of a week is recommended.

- Eat plenty of the foods that you are testing. Have at least two good helpings a day or the quantity specified in the reintroduction list. If after the last test day there are no ill-effects you may assume that the food is safe to eat and therefore you can include it as normal in your diet.
- If you have a reaction stop eating the food you are testing immediately. The time it takes to recover from a reaction varies. Do not test any new foods until you are completely well again; otherwise it will be difficult to tell if any symptoms experienced are due to the new food or left over from the previous food. Do not try to rush through the list of foods – the more haste, the less speed. The average reintroduction time is two months; it will be longer if you react to several foods.
- The time it takes for symptoms to show also varies. Do not expect symptoms to develop immediately after eating a food. It may take twenty-four to forty-eight hours for a reaction to show. Sometimes symptoms appear so slowly that they are hardly noticeable to begin with. This is why it is important to keep a diary – you can look back and see when you were last really well and this will help you spot the offending food.
- Drink plenty of water to help recover from a reaction. Some people find that adding a little bicarbonate of soda increases the effectiveness of this treatment. If you need any painkillers, take only the soluble preparations of paracetamol or Solpadeine.
- Some foods are made up of more than one ingredient. These ingredients will need to be tested separately as if a reaction occurs, you will not know which ingredient caused it. For example, bread is made from yeast and wheat. You will need to test yeast first before you can test the wheat in bread.
- Try to introduce foods in the order that they appear in the list on pages 47–48. You may miss out a food that you never eat, but if it is included as an ingredient of another food that you eat you should still test it. For example, you

may not eat a boiled or fried egg, but you may consume an egg as a cake ingredient. Foods eaten only occasionally can be moved to the end of the list, but do not forget to test them. If you suspect a food upsets you, you should still test it in case you have identified it wrongly.

- Take a week to test wheat, as symptoms often develop slowly and may be missed. For the first four days test white wheat products such as white flour, white pasta and white bread (if yeast is tolerated). For the remaining three days try testing higher-fibre wheat products including wholemeal or granary bread and breakfast cereals such as Weetabix or Shreddies. It is wise to leave the testing of wheat until late in the reintroductions, when you have a little experience under your belt.
- Sometimes you may suspect that a food upsets you, but are not absolutely sure. Don't waste time testing and retesting one food; leave it out for a few weeks and come back to it later, when your diet is less restricted.
- At the end of the reintroductions you must go back and retest all foods you believe affect you. Some suspected reactions may have been coincidental and some food intolerances rapidly disappear. There is no point in avoiding a food unless you really have to.

Order of food reintroduction

Test each food for two days. Test at least **twice** per day or as indicated below.

Tap water   – take throughout the day
Potatoes   – e.g. baked, boiled, mashed (without dairy products)
Milk   – 450 ml (1 pint) throughout the day
Yeast   – take three Brewers' Yeast tablets (one with each meal) or two teaspoons fresh yeast spread on the rice cakes, each day

Tea	– take at least twice per day
Rye	– test Ryvita or rye bread (check bread is wheat-free), only test rye bread if yeast was negative
Beef	– e.g. have cold slices at lunch and steak, roast or mince in the evening
Butter or margarine	– e.g. spread on rice cakes, add to potato
Onions	– test cooked and raw
Eggs	– test two per day
Oats	– test porridge, oatcakes, flapjacks
Coffee	– test coffee beans and instant coffee
Chocolate	– test plain chocolate or cocoa
Citrus fruits	– test oranges, grapefruit, satsumas, etc., or orange juice
Corn	– test Cornflakes, cornflour, sweetcorn
Cheese	– try 60g (2 oz) twice a day
White wine	– test two glasses. If yeast is not tolerated, test spirits
Yoghurt	– test two small cartons a day
Wheat	– test for seven days taking wheat at each meal (see note on page 47 on how to test wheat)
Nuts	– try different varieties, 60g (2 oz) twice a day
Barley	– test barley flakes, pearl barley
Vinegar	– e.g. test on chips or in salad dressing

Frequently asked questions

Will my diet be nutritionally balanced?

Hopefully, you will need to avoid only one or two foods and will find your diet reasonably straightforward. If you are avoiding a number of foods, or a few important ones such as milk or wheat, ask your doctor to refer you to a dietitian to check that your diet is nutritionally balanced and to get ideas on replacement foods.

Try to eat a wide range of your safe foods rather than restricting yourself to a few. Check that you are following the guidelines for a balanced diet, outlined on page 63. If you are milk- and dairy product-intolerant you may not be getting enough calcium in your diet. Choose a calcium-enriched soya milk and include non-dairy sources of calcium in your diet such as tofu (soya bean curd), soya cheese, tinned fish (with bones), seeds, nuts, dried fruit, pulses, green vegetables and white bread. You may require a calcium supplement such as calcium gluconate or calcium carbonate, available from chemists. Discuss this with your doctor or dietitian.

If you are avoiding a number of foods you may benefit from a multivitamin or a multivitamin and mineral supplement such as Centrum, Sanatogen Gold or Forceval. Again, discuss this with your doctor or dietitian and check that the supplement is free of any ingredients that upset you, such as wheat, yeast, corn or milk. It is inadvisable to take large doses of individual vitamins and minerals as these are wasted if they exceed the amount required by the body and may even be toxic.

Will I be able to eat the foods that upset me again?

A reliable way to rid people of their food intolerances has not yet been found. Several methods have been tried, such as administering small quantities of the food as drops under the tongue or as an injection into the skin (known as enzyme-potentiated desensitization). Various drugs have also been tried. However, these have all produced disappointing results. We are now investigating whether supplementing the diet with various types of healthy bacteria can correct the fermentation of foods in the bowel. This is still in experimental stages. For now, while the intolerance continues, you will have to resign yourself to excluding the upsetting foods – as long as that seems preferable to suffering the symptoms.

However, many people find that after avoiding a food for several months it no longer upsets them, so recheck your food intolerances periodically – every six months, say – and you may be pleasantly surprised.

Could I develop more food intolerances ?

Intolerances can change; just as intolerances can disappear, occasionally new ones can develop. Operations, courses of antibiotics, virus infections and bouts of gastroenteritis are some of the reasons for this happening. It may be easy for you to identify a food that has brought back your symptoms but if not, you will need to take yourself through the basic two-week diet and testing again.

What should I do if I have many food intolerances ?

If you are unlucky and find that a large number of foods upset you, you should think seriously about whether it's worth trying to control your symptoms by diet. You should certainly ask your doctor to refer you to a dietitian who can check the nutritional value of what you are eating, and you should discuss other ways of coping with your symptoms with your doctor. If it is agreed that you can safely continue controlling your symptoms by diet rather than with drugs, it may help if you rotate your diet. We have found that when people can eat only a few foods, they eat so much of them that they may later get into trouble with these foods as well. Rotating your diet means that you eat foods from each food group only every three or four days, so that you are not overexposed to any.

Below is an example of a rotating diet; you will obviously have to adapt it according to your particular intolerances. Check the recipe section for ideas on how to make interesting and varied meals from the foods listed.

	Day 1	Day 2	Day 3
Carbohydrate	rice, potato	millet, sweet potato	sago, buckwheat
Protein	poultry, beef	lamb, pulses	pork, fish
Vegetable	carrots, broccoli	parsnip, green beans	salad, courgette
Fruit	melon, pear	apple, mango	banana, pineapple

Common problems

Hunger!

If you are feeling hungry on the exclusion diet, it is probably because you are not replacing the foods you normally eat with suitable alternatives. In particular, you may not be eating enough of the starchy carbohydrate foods. Bread and potatoes are the main sources of starch in the British diet and without these you may have difficulty in satisfying your appetite. It is very important that you substitute these with alternative starchy carbohydrates at each meal. For example, breakfast should include rice cereal, rice cakes or one of the suggestions in the breakfast recipe section. For lunch, try a rice or buckwheat pasta salad or check the recipe section on snack lunches for some other ideas. Sweet potatoes are a good alternative to potatoes for your evening meal. Other substitutes for potato are listed on page 54. It is helpful always to have a home-made cake or biscuit (see recipes in baking section) at hand to silence a hungry stomach.

Losing weight

It is fairly common to lose a few pounds while on the exclusion diet, and for some this is an added bonus! A few people find they lose a lot of weight over a short period of time, which is likely to be due to fluid loss. Fluid retention can be a symptom of food intolerance and once the food or foods responsible are removed from the diet, the extra fluid is lost rapidly.

However, if you do not wish to lose weight or if you are losing weight too quickly, you will need to make some adjustments to your diet. Make sure you are having at least three substantial meals each day and include snacks (see recipes in baking section) in between. Try to follow the meal guidelines given on page 63. Increase your portion sizes of the carbohydrate foods such as rice, rice noodles and sweet potatoes, and of the protein foods (meat, fish and pulses) at both lunch and your evening meal. Try not to fill up on fruit and vegetables, since these will supply few calories. Include puddings regularly. Add milk-free margarine to rice cakes and sweet potatoes and use suitable oils to stir-fry meat and vegetables.

Tiredness

You may feel tired during the first few days of the diet, especially if you are used to drinking large amounts of coffee and tea, as these are stimulants. It is advisable to take things easy at the start of the diet. If the tiredness continues, it may be because you are not eating enough. In particular, you may need to eat more of the carbohydrate foods, as discussed above, which help to sustain your energy levels. If you are following the meal guidelines given on page 63 your diet should be well balanced and you should not need to take any extra vitamins or minerals. However, if you wish, you may take a multivitamin to see if this helps improve your energy levels. You should check that this supplement is free of wheat, corn or potato starch, and also milk and yeast. If you still feel tired you should ask your doctor to check whether you are anaemic.

Headaches

These are also common during the first few days of the diet, particularly if you are used to drinking a lot of coffee or tea. Try to avoid taking any painkillers, but if necessary use a soluble preparation such as soluble paracetamol or Solpadeine. If headaches continue make sure that you are drinking enough fluids (aim for ten cups or glasses a day) and that you are eating regular meals and snacks with carbohydrate-rich foods.

Worsening symptoms

You should find that you steadily improve during the second week of the diet. If your symptoms become worse, it is possible that you are intolerant to one of the foods normally found to be safe. If the symptoms are continual, the offending food is likely to be one which you are including daily, such as soya products or rice. You should try a few days without the suspected food to see if there is an improvement. If you do not feel any better, reintroduce that food and continue for a few more days, avoiding a different food. Another consideration is whether you are eating more fruit, vegetables or pulses (peas, beans and lentils) than normal, as too much fibre may trigger symptoms. If your symptoms are intermittent you should check through your diary for foods eaten within the previous twenty-four hours. Compare the foods you recorded with the list of foods on page 40. Foods that upset 10 to 20 per cent of patients are the most likely to be the cause. If you have eaten one of these you should avoid it and include it in the list of foods to test at the end of the two weeks.

Constipation

If you are used to eating wholegrain breakfast cereals and wholemeal bread you may find your fibre intake is lower on the exclusion diet, resulting in constipation. You will need to replace this fibre with other sources of fibre such as fruit, vegetables, pulses and grains such as millet and buckwheat. Constipation may also be a result of a reduced fluid intake. Make sure you replace the cups of tea and coffee you used to drink with similar amounts of other drinks. If the constipation does not resolve you may need to consider taking a bulking agent (see page 36). You should discuss the problem with your doctor.

Bloating and wind

In contrast, an increase in bloating and wind suggests you are eating too much fruit and vegetables, perhaps because you are struggling to find enough foods on the diet to fill up on. Try to keep to a maximum of two portions of fruit and two portions of vegetables (in addition to sweet potato) a day. Avoid pulses, dried fruit and brassicas (broccoli, cauliflower, cabbage and Brussels sprouts). If you find you need to eat high-fibre foods to prevent constipation, you may benefit from taking a bulking agent (see page 36).

Eating out

Eating out in the early stages of an exclusion diet is virtually impossible, unless the chef is particularly helpful. Similarly, all take-aways should be avoided. If it is difficult to avoid going out for a meal, keep to plain meat or fish, vegetables and rice (or potato once this has been introduced). Avoid sauces and eat fruit as a starter and dessert. If you eat a food that is not on the safe diet be prepared for symptoms the following day. You may need to delay reintroducing any foods for a few days until the symptoms have disappeared.

Experimenting with new foods

If you discover that you have food intolerances you cannot expect your diet to be just the same as ever, any more than you would expect food to be the same abroad as it is at home. You will have to be willing to experiment a little and get used to new tastes and textures. There are many substitutes for all the common ingredients such as potato, wheat and milk.

Alternatives to potatoes

Good alternatives to potatoes are the starchy root vegetables listed below. Other root vegetables such as swede, parsnip and turnip have a lower starch content and, although a valuable part of the diet, especially if combined with grains (see below), will not be as filling.

Sweet potatoes, which are yellow, orange or red in colour, are excellent potato substitutes, because they are very starchy and can be boiled, mashed, baked or fried in the same way as potatoes. They can usually be found in supermarkets. If you are boiling them, add a little lemon juice to the water to prevent discolouring (provided your diet permits it). Sweet potatoes are very good mashed and flavoured with cinnamon or nutmeg.

Yams have a faint nutty flavour. Cook and serve as for sweet potato. Yam flour is high in starch and can be used in casseroles, soups and for baking.

Eddoes or **taros** are eaten in the Pacific Islands and in parts of Africa and Asia. They have similar nutritional properties to potato and yam.

Cassava and **plantain** are other, less easily available substitutes for potato. These are staple foods eaten in some parts of South America, Africa and Asia.

Alternatively, potatoes can be replaced with rice or rice pasta or any of the grains listed below (without an asterix).

Alternative grains and flours

The gluten in flours used for baking is elastic and holds air. This is why a strong (high-gluten) wheat flour is ideal for bread-making. Flours made from grains that are suitable for people with wheat intolerance are less likely to rise and great patience is needed to master the skills of baking (we give advice in the recipe section on baking).

Commercial gluten-free flours usually contain either wheat or corn starch. Therefore, if you are intolerant to either of these cereals, these flours will be unsuitable. They also tend to be very expensive.

Most of the flours listed are obtainable from wholefood or health-food shops, or may be milled from the grains in a powerful domestic blender. These are cheapest if bought in bulk from wholefood retailers. Best results are usually obtained by combining flours with different properties, as described below. **Flours that are not suitable for the initial two weeks of the exclusion diet are marked with an asterix.**

Amaranth is an ancient grain originating from Mexico. It is in fact a seed which is ground into flour. High in protein, calcium and iron, it is best combined with a high-starch flour such as tapioca or potato for baking. It has a nutty flavour. Puffed amaranth may be used as a breakfast cereal. Unfortunately, amaranth is becoming increasingly difficult to obtain in the UK.

Arrowroot is a starchy root with the consistency of cornflour. It is almost pure starch, providing little besides carbohydrate, and is most useful as a thickening agent for gravies and sauces.

Buckwheat is confusingly named, as it is unrelated to wheat and therefore perfectly safe to eat for those with wheat intolerance. The grain can be bought either roasted or unroasted, the roasted being stronger in flavour. Put the buckwheat into four times its volume of cold salted water, bring to the boil and simmer until the buckwheat is soft (about fifteen minutes). Do not stir while cooking. The flour, which has a strong and distinctive flavour, has an egg-like binding capacity which makes it very good in batters. It contains some protein and is rich in B vitamins and fibre. Some buckwheat products, for example spaghetti, are sold ready-made. Read the labels with special care as some also contain wheat flour.

Carob flour is ground from the pod of the locust tree and has a strong chocolate taste. As well as being high in pectin, it contains appreciable amounts of protein, carbohydrate, calcium and phosphorous. It is an invaluable alternative to chocolate for flavouring cakes and drinks.

*Chestnut flour** is derived from the sweet chestnut. It has a distinctive flavour and is rather heavy, but can be used for baking cakes and biscuits (for example, shortbread, scones and fruit crumbles).

Gram flour is made from ground chickpeas and is therefore high in fibre. It is widely used in Indian breads and batters and is high in protein, vitamins and minerals. It has a strong flavour and will become bitter if kept too long.

*****Maize** (or **cornflour**) is a good thickening agent. It may be used in cakes, biscuits and bread, or for the Italian dish, polenta.

Millet, like rice, is a member of the grass family, but both are distant enough relatives of wheat to be safe for many people with wheat intolerance. It has good nutritional value, providing B vitamins, minerals and protein. Millet is available as a grain, flake or flour. It can be used in a variety of sweet and savoury dishes. Cook as for buckwheat. In some savoury dishes millet can be dry roasted in the pan first to enhance the flavour.

*****Potato flour,** sometimes called fecule or farina, is an excellent thickening agent and is useful for baking when mixed with other flours. It is a pure starch with little flavour of its own. (Instant mashed potato is not a pure potato flour and should not be used as a substitute.)

Quinoa is a seed which can be used as a substitute for rice in savoury or sweet dishes. It has a mild nutty flavour. Originating from South America, it is high in protein, E and B vitamins and fibre. Before cooking, rinse thoroughly in cold water. Then cook as for rice for about ten minutes or according to instructions.

Rice flour, rice flakes and ground rice can be used for baking cakes and making puddings. Rice flour is best mixed with other flours as it has a strong flavour.

Sago flour is like rice flour in texture but comes from the trunk of the palm tree. It is almost pure starch with no strong flavour. It is good for making puddings and thickening stews.

Sorghum is a type of millet commonly eaten in Africa, North India and China. It is a good source of protein, calcium and iron. It may be used to make porridge or cooked as rice. The flour can be used in cakes or flatbreads.

Soya flour is made from ground soya beans. It is a good source of protein and B vitamins and is the only pulse to contain significant amounts of fat. It has a strong flavour and is best used in combination with other flours.

Tapioca comes from the root of the tropical plant, cassava. Like sago, it is almost pure starch. It can be used by itself to make a pudding, but it is also handy for thickening soups and stews. Cassava flour (or manioc) is usually coarser and may be blended with other flours to make bread.

Varieties of wheat

The following grains are all forms of wheat and are therefore not suitable for an exclusion, gluten-free or wheat-free diet.

Bulgar is an ancient wheat that survived in Eastern Europe and is now eaten in many parts of the world. It is usually sold as cooked, parboiled wheat. It has a good taste and nutritional content.

Couscous is derived from semolina, which is a wheat product. A staple food of North Africa now readily available in Britain, it makes a good alternative to pasta, rice or potato.

Cracked wheat is made by splitting the hard outer casing of the grain. This retains its nutritional value while enabling it to cook faster.

Kibbled wheat is formed when the whole grain is cracked into little pieces rather than milled. It is used in bread-making and in breakfast cereals.

Semolina is a wheat product and should not be confused with short-grain rice, tapioca or sago.

Spelt and **Kamut** are ancient grains which have not been altered genetically over the years. Some people find they are able to tolerate these better than wheat, but they contain gluten and are not suitable for coeliacs.

Triticale is a man-made grain formed by crossing wheat and rye to improve nutritional value. It can be used to make bread.

Alternatives to dairy products

Soya milk is made from soya beans and may be obtained from health-food shops or supermarkets. Unopened, it does not need refrigeration, but after opening it should be kept in the refrigerator and used within three days. Soya milk can be used in cooking in the same way as cow's milk. Hot drinks should be allowed to cool slightly before adding soya milk to prevent it from separating. Soya milk is naturally low in calcium, but some brands are enriched with this mineral and are therefore a better substitute for cow's milk. These are usually sweetened with apple juice or fruit sugar.

There are a large number of useful soya products available, such as soya margarine, cheese, yoghurt, ice-creams and other desserts. These are all suitable for a milk-free diet but may contain ingredients not allowed on the exclusion diet and therefore labels should be checked carefully. Tofu is soya bean curd. It is high in protein and calcium and a good meat substitute for vegetarians. It is available plain or smoked. Plain varieties quickly absorb the flavour of a marinade and when stir-fried have a similar texture to chicken. Do not mistake Quorn for tofu. Quorn is made from a microfungus which is a relative of the mushroom and another good meat substitute. However, it contains egg white and is therefore not suitable for the initial stage of the exclusion diet.

Rice milks are also available in most health-food shops. They are made from brown rice and may have oil, salt and flavourings added. Nutritionally, they are not a good substitute for milk, but they are useful in expanding the diet if soya milk is not tolerated. *Oat milks* and *pea milks* are also now available.

Goat's and **sheep's milk,** cheese and yoghurt may be tested if cow's milk is not tolerated. However, they are similar in nature to cow's milk and should be avoided on the first stage of the exclusion diet. Some people with cow's milk intolerance find that after a while they also become intolerant of goat's and sheep's milk.

Spreading and cooking fats. Being a cow's milk product, butter is not allowed on exclusion and milk-free diets. Most margarines also contain milk and should be avoided. Margarines that are 100 per cent dairy-free include soya and sunflower varieties. They can be found in health-food shops and some supermarkets. Some varieties contain vegetable oils, which may or may not include corn (or maize) oil. This should be checked with the manufacturer (some addresses are given at the end of the book) to determine whether a margarine is suitable for the exclusion diet. Commercial vegetable oil is a blend of oils and usually contains corn. This should be avoided on the exclusion diet and replaced with, for example, sunflower, olive, rapeseed or safflower oils.

Egg substitutes. It is possible to replace eggs in recipes with commercial egg replacers. Although these have little nutritional value, they can be very useful in cooking. Check the ingredients carefully to determine whether they are suitable for the exclusion diet. Other substitutes for eggs in cooking are given in the introduction of the recipe section.

Alternative savoury flavourings

Miso is a fermented mixture of cereal grains, soya beans, water and salt. The form containing rice will be suitable for many people with food intolerance, but be careful not to confuse it with other varieties containing wheat or barley. Miso is rich in protein, minerals and vitamins, including vitamin B_{12}. It has a thick, pasty consistency and is thinned with water (but not boiling water, as this curdles it) to be used as a stock base in soups, stews, sauces and gravies.

Tahini is made from sesame seeds crushed and blended with oil. It is useful for making sauces and in the dip, hummus. For people who do not tolerate lemon, an added amount of garlic and parsley makes an excellent alternative. Tahini can also be included in salad dressing or spread on rice cakes.

Tamari is a wheat-free soya sauce. It is a useful flavouring in savoury dishes such as stir-fries and to enhance the flavour of gravy.

Gravy mixes usually contain yeast and wheat or corn starch. There are some gravy brownings available (e.g. Burdell's or Crosse and Blackwell's) that contain caramel and salt only and these can be added to meat juices to provide colour. Some health-food shops supply wheat- and yeast-free gravy mixes, but check the rest of the ingredients carefully.

Creamed coconut or **coconut milk** are useful ingredients, particularly in Chinese or Thai style dishes. They may be used in both savoury and sweet sauces.

Mirrin is a sweet Japanese seasoning, suitable for the exclusion diet. It is available from good health food shops and is useful in marinades and stir-fries. In some recipes it can be replaced with sweet rice vinegar.

Further suggestions for gravies, sauces and stocks are given in the relevant recipe section.

Alternative drinks

Cutting out tea and coffee offers a chance to experiment with a variety of alternative drinks. There is a wide range of herbal and fruit teas to choose from (avoid those with added citrus peel) as well as flavoured soya milks and fruit juices.

Camomile tea or hot carob-flavoured soya milk are relaxing at bedtime. Use the carob flour like cocoa powder. Earlier in the day, peppermint tea or pineapple juice are refreshing. Rooibosh herbal tea is the closest in taste to normal tea. Chicory is a good alternative to coffee and the ground variety can be brewed in the same way as ground coffee. Soya milk shakes can be made at home by liquidizing fresh or tinned fruit with soya milk, or you can buy them from health-food shops. For a change, try a mixture of apple and grape juice with ice and a sprig of mint, or tomato juice with a touch of paprika.

The recipe section on beverages gives some more ideas for new drinks to try.

A sample menu

The simple guidelines below are intended to help make sure that the exclusion diet you are following is nutritionally balanced. You can exchange the foods listed with ideas from the relevant recipe sections in this book. For a main meal you may wish to add a soup or starter and in between meals you can try suggestions in the baking section. There are also recipe ideas for packed lunches and snacks, desserts and special occasions.

If you are hoping to lose weight on the exclusion diet, cut down on both fats and sugars. Do not fry foods, use only a scraping of margarine on rice cakes and do not use it on vegetables or add oily dressings to salads. Try to avoid sugary foods such as cakes and puddings; eat fresh fruit or fruit-based dishes instead.

If you are underweight, make desserts part of your meals and eat snacks in between. You should also have large portions of rice, sweet potatoes, meat and fish. Try to include plenty of soya products such as soya milk (as drinks and on cereal), soya yoghurt and other soya desserts.

Breakfast	Rice Krispies, soya milk and sugar Rice cakes, milk-free margarine and jam Apple juice/herbal tea
Snack meal	Meat/poultry/ fish Cold rice salad or rice cakes Salad Fruit/soya yoghurt Ribena
Main meal	Meat/poultry/fish Sweet potato/rice/buckwheat pasta/rice noodles Vegetables Fruit- or soya-based dessert Herbal tea

Nutritional supplements

Vitamins and minerals

If your diet is varied and well balanced it is unlikely that you will need extra vitamins and minerals. If you are concerned that your diet is limited, ask your doctor to refer you to a state-registered dietitian who can recommend alternative foods rich in the nutrients you may be lacking or, if necessary, a suitable supplement. In some cases, individual vitamins or minerals may be necessary, e.g. calcium for those on a dairy-free diet.

If you are considering taking a supplement it is generally advisable to take a multivitamin or a multivitamin and mineral as a single tablet or capsule rather than large doses of individual vitamins and minerals. This is for several reasons :

• Water-soluble vitamins (vitamins B and C) are eliminated in the urine if they exceed the body's requirements. These vitamins are therefore wasted if taken in large doses.

- Some vitamins are toxic if taken in excessive quantities, e.g. vitamins A, D and B_6.
- Overdosing on single minerals may affect the absorption of others. Very high intakes of calcium or iron, for instance, can reduce absorption of zinc.
- Taking a combination of single, high dose minerals and vitamins is much more expensive than taking a single combined supplement.

Health supplements

There are a large number of 'health' supplements available that claim to ease a wide range of symptoms and ailments. However, few (if any) scientific trials have been performed to date to substantiate these claims. These supplements tend to be very expensive. If you wish to try a product but do not notice any improvement in your health after a few weeks, we suggest that you do not continue using it.

Probiotics

A probiotic is a live bacterial supplement which improves the intestinal microbial balance. To date, probiotics are available in this country either as an ingredient in bioyoghurts or in the form of powders, tablets or liquid preparations. These preparations contain a variety of different strains of bacteria, mainly lactobacilli, streptococci and bifidobacter.

For a probiotic to be effective a significant quantity has to reach the lower bowel. In some commercial preparations it is questionable whether many of the organisms survive the passage through the intestines. The probiotic needs to be taken every day because it appears to be difficult for the microbes to permanently attach themselves to the bowel. Once treatment stops, any beneficial effects wear off.

Our own studies indicate that a proportion of patients with irritable bowel syndrome improve when treated with probiotics while the treatment lasts. Some strains of bacteria appear to be more effective than others, but this varies between patients. Probiotics can be particularly helpful in restoring the balance of bacteria in the bowel after treatment with antibiotics or a gastrointestinal infection.

If you wish to try a probiotic supplement our advice would be to use a preparation recommended by a specialist and to take this daily, initially for a four-week period. If you do not notice an improvement in symptoms there is probably little point in continuing beyond this.

Prebiotics

A prebiotic is a non-digestible food ingredient that has a beneficial effect on health by selectively stimulating the growth and activity of one or a limited number of bacteria in the bowel. The most common source of prebiotics is the fructo-oligosaccharides which occur naturally in many fruit and vegetables such as chicory, artichokes, bananas, leeks, onions and asparagus. However, the amounts present are small and require extraction and concentration to exert an effect. Prebiotics have already been incorporated into yoghurts and there is the potential for a wider use in common foods such as cereals and confectionery for consumption as part of a normal diet.

Studies on healthy volunteers have shown that prebiotics are able to increase the proportion of healthy bacteria in the gut. We have studied the effect of prebiotic supplements on patients with irritable bowel syndrome. Unfortunately, no significant change in patients' symptoms was detected, although further clinical studies are required.

THE RECIPES

Introduction

An exclusion diet need not be repetitive and boring. The recipes in the following sections were designed by Pamela Harris, who has been on a restricted diet herself for the past seven years and has gained a wealth of experience in creating delicious dishes.

Cooking with unfamiliar foods may appear daunting at first, but with patience and practice you may well be surprised with the results. These tips from Pamela should help make your new style of cooking both enjoyable and successful:

- If you are unable to find an ingredient that appears in these recipes in your local supermarket or health-food shop, check the specialist suppliers (see pages 186–188) for availability. Chinese and Indian supermarkets and delicatessens are also good places to look and are often much cheaper. Buy a small amount initially, but if you find the products useful, order in bulk later to save money. The same ingredients have been used in a number of different recipes to minimize any waste.

- Try to build up some store-cupboard ingredients, such as:

rice noodles	pumpkin seeds	banana chips
ground rice	sunflower seeds	dried apricots
arrowroot	pine nuts (not true nuts)	dried mango
pulses and beans	desiccated coconut	dried pineapple
spices		

- Buy fresh herbs in pots and use over two to three days. Continue to water the pot and you should get a second growth. Put any leftovers in the freezer. Herb oils are excellent and have a long shelf life. Buy a large bottle of your supermarket's own brand of sunflower oil. Decant into smaller bottles and add plenty of herbs, for example, lemon thyme or marjoram. Seal the bottles and let them stand for at least a month before using.

- Keep all alternative flours in the refrigerator to prolong their freshness.

- When making bread, make two loaves at a time and keep spare slices and a bag of breadcrumbs in the freezer. A bag of frozen home-made cake crumbs is also very useful.

- Wheat-free flours are lighter than normal flour and therefore less fat is needed than in standard recipes.

- Wheat-free products require a lower temperature and a longer cooking time. Refrigerating the dough for twenty to thirty minutes before baking helps improve the flavour and texture. Use smaller dishes and tins, greasing them very well.

- Home-made stock has the best flavour and is the most economical (see page 143). Buy cheap offcuts of meat from your butcher and boil them with vegetables and herbs to make a stock. If cooking for one or two people, freeze it in an ice-cube tray. For convenience, you can also use some of the commercial products that are available. Supermarkets offer their own fresh stocks, although chicken stock tends to be the only one suitable for the exclusion diet (check the ingredients carefully). Some stock cubes and powders available from health-food shops are wheat-, dairy- and yeast-free.

- When buying meat, especially cubed, look in supermarket freezer cabinets, which stock lean, economically priced packs of beef, lamb, pork and chicken.

- Sugar in recipes can be replaced with honey or a concentrated syrupy fruit juice. However, remember that these contain more moisture and you may not need to add as much liquid as the recipe suggests. Fruit sugar, or fructose, may also be used in place of sugar. In general, reduce the amount in recipe by a quarter.

- Soya cream works well in recipes and is reasonably heat stable. Check ingredients are suitable for your diet.

- Check when buying spices that these are wheat-free.

- In most pasta dishes, pasta can be replaced with rice or rice noodles.

- For those who have problems with eggs, here are some tips:

  Use unflavoured vegetable gelatine instead (1 tsp dry gelatine to 2 tbsp liquid for each egg).

  Substitute mashed banana, apricot purée or puréed vegetables (2 tbsp for each egg).

  Various egg replacers are on the market. Check carefully, as most contain whey powder.

- Electrical kitchen equipment, e.g. blenders, liquidizers and food processors, make life a lot easier. You will need to add less liquid using this equipment than if you are mixing by hand. Add liquid gradually to prevent the mixture from becoming too heavy – you will learn to find the right consistency through experience.

- Finally, do not expect too much too quickly. Read as much as you can about the ingredients you are using and scan cookery books for ideas. You will soon find you can select information that relates to you and customize recipes to suit your requirements.

Symbols

The recipes in this book are, as far as possible, free from artificial colourings, flavourings and preservatives. They are also free from gluten (wheat, rye and barley), wheat starch, oats, cow's milk and corn (apart from some of the flour mixes used in the baking section). If you simply want to exclude one or more of these from your diet you may choose any recipe you wish. If you are following the first stage of the exclusion diet, the exclusion diet for arthritis or are excluding eggs you should select only those appropriately marked (see below). If other foods are to be excluded you will need to examine the list of ingredients in each recipe carefully to see whether it is suitable for your diet.

The symbols used in this book for the special diets are:

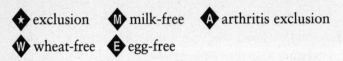

Measurements

Measurements are given in both metric and imperial units. Use one system only; do not combine them.

Where spoonfuls are referred to, level spoons are meant unless otherwise stated.

    1 tsp (teaspoon) = 5 ml
    1 tbsp (tablespoon) = 15 ml

To ensure success, check the size of the spoons you are using. Australian readers should remember that as their tablespoon has been converted to 20 ml, and is therefore larger than the British tablespoon, they should use three 5 ml teaspoons where instructed to use one 15 ml tablespoon.

BREAKFASTS

Breakfast cheers

Serves 1

1 small tub soya yoghurt
1 dessertspoon clear honey
6 dried apricots, poached, plus 1–2 tbsp of the poaching juice

Put all the ingredients into a blender and process to a smooth drink, adding a little more apricot juice if necessary.
Raspberries can be used in place of apricots to vary the flavour.

Breakfast crunch

Serves 2

1 small tub soya yoghurt
1 tsp clear honey
1 tbsp sunflower seeds, toasted
1 tsp raisins, chopped
1 tsp dried apricots, chopped

Empty the yoghurt into a sundae dish and drizzle with the honey. Mix together the seeds, raisins and apricots and sprinkle on top.

Winter warmer breakfast

Serves 2

60 g/2 oz mixture of rice and millet flakes
200 ml/¹/₃ pint water
2 tsp clear honey (to taste)
1 level tbsp dried apricots
1 level tbsp mixture of sultanas, raisins or chopped dates

Put the flakes and water in a saucepan, bring to the boil and simmer for 3–4 minutes. Remove from the heat and stir in the honey, apricots and other fruit of choice.

Pan-fried herring roes

Serves 1

115 g/4 oz herring roes
30 g/1 oz dairy-free margarine plus 1 tsp sunflower oil
little rice vinegar
salt and pepper

Put the roes in a basin, cover with water and add 1 dessert-spoon of rice vinegar. Leave for 10 minutes to clean. Drain and rinse the roes in fresh cold water and pat dry.

Put the oil and margarine in a shallow pan and heat gently; do not allow the margarine to brown. Lay the roes in the pan, season and cook gently for about 6–7 minutes, depending on thickness, turning once.

Remove the roes, drain on kitchen paper and transfer to a plate. Keep warm.

If necessary, add a little fresh margarine to the juices in pan. Add 1 tsp rice vinegar (or to taste). Add parsley and stir together. Spoon the juices over the roes and serve.

Zingy mushrooms

Serves 1

2 large flat mushrooms
1 heaped tbsp rice, preferably brown, cooked
1 medium tomato, skinned and chopped
1 tsp wheat-free Worcester sauce, or to taste
1/2 tbsp wheat-free mustard
small knob dairy-free margarine
salt and pepper

Wipe the mushrooms clean. Mix together the rice and tomato, season lightly and add the Worcester sauce and mustard. Mix well.

Spread the mixture over the mushrooms and dot the top with a small knob of margarine.

Bake at 180°C/350°F/Gas Mark 4 for 15–20 minutes.

Bacon rosti brunch

Serves 1

115 g/4 oz unsmoked streaky bacon, de-rinded and chopped
115 g/4 oz sweet potatoes, coarsely grated
115 g/4 oz cabbage, finely shredded
1 egg, beaten
1 tsp rice or millet flour mix
2 spikes chives, chopped
salt and pepper

Put the bacon, potatoes and cabbage in a bowl and season to taste. Stir in the flour and chives, add the egg and mix well.

Heat a little oil in frying pan, drop in spoonfuls of mixture, and fry for about 7–8 minutes, turning once.

Drain on kitchen paper and serve with grilled tomatoes.

Pear to please

Serves 1

1 large fresh pear
1 heaped tbsp ready-to-eat prunes, minced
1 tbsp pure apricot preserve
toasted pine nuts (optional)

Peel and halve the pear, gently removing the core.

Mix the prunes with the apricot preserve and fill the pear.

Sprinkle with the toasted pine nuts if desired.

Honeyed banana bread

Serves 1

2 slices wheat-free soda bread (see page 160)
1 banana
1 tbsp clear honey, warmed
pinch cinnamon

Wrap the soda bread slices loosely in tin foil. Put in the oven to slightly warm through. Remove from the oven and place on a warm plate.

Mash the banana and add the warm honey. Spread over the slices of bread and lightly dust with cinnamon.

Raisin start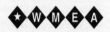

Serves 2

1/2 cup seedless raisins
2 ripe pears
1 small tub soya yoghurt
little cinnamon (to taste)

Soak the raisins in just enough hot water to cover for 15–20 minutes, until plump and moist. Meanwhile, peel and core the pears and cut into chunks.

Put the yoghurt in a blender, drain the raisins and add to the blender along with the pears. Blend together until fairly smooth.

Pour into individual dishes and sprinkle with cinnamon to taste.

PACKED LUNCHES AND SNACKS

Savoury scones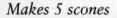

Makes 5 scones

225 g/8 oz flour mix and 2 tsp wheat-free baking powder
   (see page 158)
pinch salt
60 g/2 oz dairy-free margarine
2 tbsp chopped ham
1 tbsp chopped sundried tomato (dried of any oil)
2 tsp basil leaves, torn
1/2 tsp wheat-free Dijon mustard
3–4 tbsp soya milk
1 egg, beaten

Sift the flour and baking powder into a bowl and add the salt. Rub in the margarine to a breadcrumb consistency, then stir in the ham, tomatoes and basil. Thoroughly mix the mustard into the milk. Add the egg to the mixture and sufficient milk to make a fairly stiff but not too sticky dough. Roll out and cut into 5 buns. Brush the tops with a little extra milk and bake for 10–12 minutes (do not over-bake) at 200°C/400°F/Gas Mark 5.

As a variation, the ham, tomato and basil can be replaced with chicken, chives and sweet pepper.

Savoury tarts

Makes 6 individual or 6 slices

wheat-free shortcrust pastry using 170g (6oz) flour mix (see
    page 158)
450 ml (3/4 pint) white sauce (see page 145)

Choice of filling:

    (a) prawn, parsley and chopped cucumber
    (b) flaked tuna and broccoli
    (c) chopped cooked chicken and mushroom
    (d) cooked minced beef, tomato purée and a little ginger
    (e) chopped ham, green pepper and pineapple

Line a greased flan dish with the pastry or use individual dishes. Stir the chosen filling into the white sauce and fill the pastry case. Bake at 200°C/400°F/Gas Mark 5 for approximately 20 minutes or until the pastry is browned.

Fruity wild rice salad

Serves 2

60 g/2 oz wild rice (raw weight), cooked
1 eating apple, chopped
1 tbsp herb dressing (see page 146)
1 large stick celery, sliced
30 g/1 oz dried apricots, chopped
1/2 mango, chopped
few sunflower seeds
few sprigs watercress

Put the rice into a bowl, stir in a little vinagrette dressing over the chopped apple and add to the rice. Fork through, adding a little more dressing if necessary. Add the celery, mango, apricots and sunflower seeds and gently mix. Serve with a garnish of watercress.

Tuna and apple salad

Serves 2

85 g/3 oz cooked brown rice
2 medium eating apples, e.g. Cox's Orange
2 tbsp herb dressing (see page 146)
200g/7 oz tin of tuna (or required amount)
60g (2 oz) bunch watercress, washed
few pine nuts

Core and slice the apples and dip in the vinagrette dressing. Mix 2 tablespoons of vinagrette dressing into the cooked rice. Divide between two plates and lay the watercress on top. Arrange portions of tuna and apple on the watercress and sprinkle the pine nuts on top.

As quick as you can

Serves 2

4 slices wheat-free soda bread (see page 160)
1 tin sardines (medium)
Heaped tbsp cucumber, peeled and chopped
Heaped tbsp chopped sweet peppers
1 tub soya yoghurt
watercress to garnish (optional)
salt and pepper

Flake the sardines, add the cucumber, peppers, salt and pepper and stir in the yoghurt.

Toast the soda bread slices, spread the sardine mixture over top and garnish with a sprig or two of watercress in the centre of each slice.

Apricot and pineapple snacks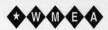

Serves 2

115 g/4 oz dried apricots
115 g/4 oz dried pineapple
115 g/4 oz desiccated coconut
1–2 tbsp white grape juice/apple juice
few drops pure almond essence (if not allowed, vanilla)
little desiccated ground coconut

Put the apricots and pineapple in a bowl, cover with boiling water, leave to stand for 20 minutes, then drain.

Put the fruit and coconut in a blender, process lightly and transfer to the bowl. Add the grape juice and almond essence and mix together. Add more juice or coconut as necessary.

Shape into balls, roll in ground coconut and place in cake papers. Place in the refrigerator to set.

VEGETARIAN DISHES

Harvest vegetable pie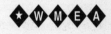

Serves 6

2 medium carrots, cubed
1 large parsnip, cut into pieces
115 g/4 oz small cauliflower florets
115 g/4 oz small broccoli florets
115 g/4 oz fine beans, cut into pieces
170 g/6 oz swede, cubed
85 g/3 oz cabbage, chopped
600–850 ml/1–1½ pints vegetable stock (see page 144)
1 sprig fresh thyme and 1 bay-leaf (or bouquet garni)
4 sweet potatoes
pinch nutmeg
arrowroot
salt and pepper

Place the carrots, parsnip, cauliflower, broccoli, beans, swede and cabbage in a large pan. Add the stock, thyme and bay-leaf. Bring to the boil and reduce the heat to a simmer for approximately 15 minutes, or until vegetables are cooked.

Scrub the sweet potatoes, cook in a pan of slightly salted water and drain.

Discard the bay-leaf. Remove the vegetables with a slotted spoon and place in an ovenproof casserole dish.

Boil the stock to reduce by half and thicken with a little arrowroot. Pour over the vegetables to moisten, but not cover them.

Skin and mash the sweet potatoes, adding the nutmeg. Spread them over the vegetables. Bake at 180°C/350°F/Gas Mark 4 until the top is golden brown.

Stuffed peppers   ◆ⓌⓂⒺ

Serves 4

4 good-sized peppers, red or green
2 tbsp sunflower oil
85 g/3 oz cooked rice, preferably brown
60 g/2 oz mushrooms, finely chopped
2 spikes chives, finely chopped
60 g/2 oz bean sprouts
85–115 g/3–4 oz water chestnuts, cut into small pieces
salt and pepper
olive oil

Heat the sunflower oil in a pan and add the chives and mush-rooms. Cook for 3–4 minutes. Add the bean sprouts and water chestnuts and cook for a further 2 minutes. Remove the pan from the heat and transfer the contents into a bowl. Add the rice, season well and mix together.

Prepare the peppers, cutting off the tops to make lids,

scoop out the seeds and core. Fill with the vegetable mixture and place the lids on top.

Brush all over with olive oil and bake at 180°C/350°F/Gas Mark 4 for about 20–25 minutes.

Peking mixed vegetables

Serves 2

3 tbsp sunflower oil
1 clove garlic
25 mm/1 in fresh ginger, peeled and sliced
salt and pepper
1 large carrot, very thinly sliced
1 green pepper, de-seeded, cored and shredded
115 g/4 oz small cauliflower florets
60 g/2 oz prepared bean sprouts
60 g/2 oz water chestnuts, cut into small pieces
170 ml/6fl oz vegetable stock (see page 144)
2 tsp Tamari (wheat-free soy sauce)
1 tsp brown sugar or honey

Heat the oil in a large pan or wok. When hot, add the garlic, ginger, salt and pepper. Cook for 1–2 minutes. Add the carrots, green pepper and cauliflower and stir fry for 3–4 minutes.

Add the bean sprouts and water chestnuts and fry for another 1–2 minutes. Stirring, add the stock, Tamari and sugar. Check the seasoning. Cover and cook for 3–4 minutes.

Remove from the heat, turn onto a warm dish and serve with prepared cooked rice noodles.

Florence tart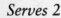

Serves 2

4 or 5 slices aubergine
170 g/6 oz wheat-free shortcrust pastry (see page 165)
2 tbsp sunflower oil
2 garlic cloves, crushed
2 large tomatoes, skinned, de-seeded and chopped
1 medium courgette, chopped
2 tsp fresh chives, chopped
salt and pepper
2 tsp fresh basil leaves, torn

Lay the aubergine slices on a plate, sprinkle with salt and leave to sweat.

Line a 15 cm/6 in flan dish or individual dishes with prepared pastry and set aside to rest. Retain pastry trimmings.

Pour the oil into a pan and lightly fry the garlic for 2–3 minutes. Add the chives and courgettes. Rinse and pat dry the aubergines, chop into small pieces and add to the pan. Cook for 4–5 minutes. Add the chopped tomatoes and cook for a further 3–4 minutes. Season to taste, add the torn basil leaves, stir and spread the mixture over the pastry case.

Roll out the pastry trimmings and cut into strips. Place over the top of the tart to make a lattice effect. Bake for approximately 20 minutes at 200°C/400°F/Gas Mark 6, or until the pastry is cooked.

Vegetable kebabs with saffron rice

Serves 3

required quantity of rice
2¹/2 times quantity of chicken stock to quantity of rice (see page 143)
pinch of saffron
pinch of cinnamon

pinch of cardomon
black pepper to taste
1 tbsp sunflower oil
1 tsp rice vinegar
1 tsp fresh thyme
1 tsp fresh rosemary
salt and pepper

Kebabs:
175 g/6 oz courgettes
6 mushrooms – 2 per person
9 cherry tomatoes – 3 per person
1 green pepper, cut into 6 pieces, 2 pieces per person
1 orange or 1 yellow pepper, cut into 6 pieces, 2 pieces per person

Mix together the oil, rice vinegar and herbs. Stir well and set aside to allow the flavours to develop. If this can be done ahead of time, so much the better.

Put the stock, saffron, cardomon and cinnamon in a pan, bring to the boil and simmer for 3–4 minutes. Wash and drain the rice and add to the pan. Stir well and cook for the required amount of time. Drain, season with black pepper, put into a heated dish and keep warm.

Heat the grill to medium, arrange the vegetables on skewers and brush well with the herb-flavoured oil. Grill the kebabs, turning and basting frequently, until cooked and lightly browned (8–10 minutes). Remove from the skewers and serve on a bed of warm rice.

Mediterranean salad with penne ◆W◆M◆E

Serves 2–3

1 avocado, sliced
340 g/12 oz fresh tomatoes, sliced
340 g/12 oz green, yellow and orange peppers, thinly sliced
black olives
280–340 g/10–12 oz rice pasta (penne variety)

Dressing:
6 tbsp olive oil
3 tbsp rice vinegar
1 tsp wheat-free Dijon mustard
1 tsp demerara sugar
1 heaped tsp fresh marjoram or basil, finely chopped

Cook the penne in lightly salted water.

Place the ingredients for the dressing in a blender or shaker, mix well and chill.

Assemble the salad ingredients, drain the penne and fold into the salad. Pour over a little dressing and sprinkle well with herbs. Serve any remaining dressing separately or refrigerate for future use.

Pasta with lentil and courgette sauce

Serves 2–3

115 g/4 oz lentils
1 tbsp sunflower oil
1 clove garlic, crushed
10 cm/4 in piece of leek, sliced
1 dessertspoon fresh chives, chopped
280 g/10 oz courgettes, chopped
400 g/14 oz tin or jar plum tomatoes
good pinch oregano
salt and pepper
340 g/12 oz rice pasta (spaghetti variety)
parsley to garnish

Soak the lentils overnight in 600 ml/1 pint of water. Simmer gently in the soaking liquid until soft.

Fry the garlic, leek and chives in oil, add the seasonings and courgettes and sauté for 10 minutes. Then add the tomatoes and lentils and cook for a further 10–15 minutes.

Cook the pasta as directed, drain and pour into a serving dish. Pour over the sauce and sprinkle with parsley.

Chilli beans hotpot

Serves 4

600 ml/1 pint vegetable stock (see page 144)
30–60g/1–2oz dairy-free margarine or sunflower oil
450 g/1 lb vegetables, e.g. swede, parsnips, carrots, celery
    and leeks, cut into small cubes
1 or 2 cloves garlic, depending on size, crushed
400 g/14 oz jar chopped tomatoes
2 heaped tbsp tomato purée
400 g/14 oz tin mixed beans (haricot, cannellini, kidney,
    etc.)
salt and pepper
chilli powder to taste
1 large sweet potato
parsley to garnish

Heat the oil in a pan and add the vegetables and garlic. Sweat for a few minutes but do not brown. Add the tomatoes, purée, seasoning and stock and stir. Add the beans and simmer over a low heat for 20–25 minutes.

Meanwhile, scrub the sweet potato well and steam or boil whole for 15–20 minutes. Drain and rinse in cold water. Slice very thinly.

Remove the beans from the heat, transfer to an ovenproof dish and adjust the seasoning as necessary.

Layer the slices of sweet potato over the beans, brush the top with oil and bake for 15–20 minutes at the top of the oven at 180°C/350°F/Gas Mark 4, or cook under the grill until browned.

Remove, sprinkle with parsley and serve.

Bean bourgignon   ◆ⓌⓂⒺ

Serves 4

1 tbsp sunflower oil
1 carrot, sliced
1 clove garlic, crushed
3 spikes chives, finely chopped
bouquet garni
$1/2$ tsp dried thyme
2 tbsp parsley, finely chopped
salt and pepper
400 g/14 oz tin red kidney beans, drained*
400 g/14 oz tin haricot beans, drained*
450 ml/$3/4$ pint vegetable stock (see page 144)
300 ml/$1/2$ pint red wine (if not allowed, increase stock)
1 tbsp tomato purée (increase to 2 tbsp if not using red wine)
1 heaped tsp soft brown sugar
60 g/2 oz dairy-free margarine
450 g/1 lb button mushrooms
$1/2$ tsp dried oregano

In a large flame-proof casserole dish, heat the oil, add the carrot, garlic and chives and fry for 6-8 minutes, stirring occasionally. Stir in the bouquet garni, thyme, parsley and season to taste.

Add both the beans, stock, wine, tomato purée and sugar. Bring to the boil, then reduce to a very low heat and simmer, covered, for 40–45 minutes.

Before the end of the cooking time, heat the margarine in a frying pan. When it is melted, add the mushrooms and oregano and fry for about 3 minutes. Using a slotted spoon, transfer the mushrooms to the casserole. Serve with boiled rice.

*Cooked fresh kidney and haricot beans can be used instead if preferred.

Asparagus stuffed pancakes

Makes 4 or 5 pancakes using a 15–18 cm/6–7 in heavy-based pan

asparagus, fresh, frozen or canned, 3 spears per pancake
85 g/3 oz flour mix (see page 158)
pinch salt
1 egg
3–4 tbsp soya milk
1 tbsp sunflower oil (preferably 'buttery' variety)
oil for cooking
2 tbsp soya cream
1/2 tsp wheat-free Dijon mustard

Steam the asparagus until it is just tender and keep warm.

Sift the flour into a bowl, add the salt and make a centre well. Add the egg and a little milk and beat with a metal spoon until smooth. Add a little more milk until a creamy consistency is reached, then add the sunflower oil. The consistency should now be a thin cream. Place in the refrigerator to rest and chill.

Brush a pan with oil and heat to a very high temperature. Beat the batter and pour in the right amount for the size of the pan. Place the pan over the heat and cook the batter, turning. When the edges are brown lift the pancake and cook the underside. When both sides are cooked, remove and keep warm.

Cook the remaining batter in the same way. Stack the pancakes with leaves of baking parchment in between to prevent them sticking together.

Stir the mustard into the cream. Place a pancake on a warmed plate and lay asparagus spears in the centre. Pour 2 tsp of the cream mixture over the asparagus and fold the pancake over. Repeat with the remaining pancakes.

Mushroom fritters ◆W◆ ◆M◆

Serves 2

115 g/4 oz mushrooms, wiped clean and finely chopped
60 g/2 oz wheat-free flour mix (see page 158)
1/2 tsp wheat-free baking powder (see page 159)
good pinch salt
1 egg
1 dessertspoon sunflower oil (preferably 'buttery' variety)
1 dessertspoon soya milk
little extra oil for frying

Mix together the flour, baking powder and salt. Stir in the chopped mushrooms.

Mix the egg with the milk, make a well in the flour mix and add the egg and milk mixture. Beat well together, add the oil and mix well.

Heat some oil in a heavy-bottomed pan. Fry a spoonful of the mixture until cooked and lightly browned, turning once. Drain on kitchen paper and serve immediately.

These fritters make a good accompaniment to a main course salad.

Butter bean curry ◆W◆ ◆M◆ ◆E◆

Serves 4

225 g/8 oz butter beans
1 tsp cumin seeds
3 tbsp sunflower oil
1 onion, chopped
30 g/1 oz fresh ginger, chopped
2 cloves garlic, crushed
1 tsp ground cumin
1 chilli, chopped
1 tsp ground coriander

1/2 tsp turmeric
4 cloves
450 g/1 lb tomatoes, skinned and chopped
2 tsp garam masala
salt and pepper

Soak the beans overnight. Then drain, rinse and cook in plenty of fresh water until tender – about 20 minutes. Drain and cover.

Dry roast the cumin seeds in a heavy-bottomed pan until they darken. Set aside.

Heat the oil in a pan and fry the onions until soft. Add the ginger and garlic and cook for 2 minutes. Add the cumin, chilli, coriander, turmeric and cloves, the tomatoes and 300 ml/1/2 pint water and cook until the tomatoes are soft. Mix with the beans and cook for a further 15 minutes.

Just before serving, stir in the garam masala and season to taste. Serve with rice.

Note: If you prefer a milder curry, omit the chilli.

Continental lentil rissoles   ★ W M E A

Serves 4

225 g/8 oz Continental lentils
2 tbsp sunflower oil
1 stick celery, chopped
1 large clove garlic, crushed
1 small green pepper, cored, seeded and chopped
1 tsp turmeric
1 tsp ground coriander
1 tsp ground cumin
1/4 tsp chilli powder
salt and pepper
rice flour for coating (use millet flour if following arthritis exclusion diet)
extra sunflower oil for frying

Soak the lentils overnight. Drain, rinse and put in a large pan with 280ml/1/2 pint of water. Bring to the boil, then simmer gently until the lentils are tender and have absorbed all the liquid – about 30–45 minutes.

Heat the oil in a pan and add the celery, garlic and green pepper. Cook for 5 minutes. Stir in the turmeric, coriander, cumin and chilli powder and cook for 2 minutes. Add the vegetable and spice mixture to the cooked lentils. Stir well and season to taste. Leave to cool.

Mould the mixture into small rissoles and coat evenly with flour. Heat some oil in a frying pan. Fry the rissoles until they are well browned and cooked through. Drain on absorbent paper before serving with brown rice and a crisp salad.

The rissoles can also be served cold.

BUDGET RECIPES

Savoury crumble   W M E

Serves 2

340 g/12 oz minced meat
1 tbsp sunflower oil
1 large carrot, chopped
1 large/2 small sticks celery, chopped
1 dessertspoon wheat-free Worcester sauce
2 tbsp tomato purée
2 tsp fresh chives
pinch thyme
150 ml/1/4 pint stock (see page 143)
salt and pepper
little arrowroot

Topping:
85 g/3 oz flour mix (see page 158 or use a mixture of rice, soya and gram flours)
40 g/11/2 oz dairy-free margarine

30 g/1 oz wheat-free breadcrumbs (see page 160)
1 tsp mixed herbs
salt and pepper

Heat the oil in a pan, add the minced meat and cook until
sealed. Then add the carrots, celery, Worcester sauce, tomato
purée, chives, thyme and stock and simmer for 15–20
minutes. Season to taste and thicken with a little arrowroot if
necessary. Turn into an ovenproof dish.

Rub the margarine into the flour, add the breadcrumbs,
mixed herbs and seasoning. Spread this crumble mix over the
meat, smooth the top and bake for 45 minutes to an hour on
180°C/350°F/Gas Mark 4.

Chicken livers with rice noodles

Serves 2

340 g/12 oz chicken livers, washed, prepared and cut into strips
115 g/4 oz unsmoked bacon pieces
2 tsp sunflower oil
60 g/2 oz mushrooms chopped
400 g/14 oz tin or jar chopped tomatoes
1/3 small green pepper, seeded, cored and chopped
2 tsp chopped dried herbs
30 g/1 oz gram flour
salt and pepper
rice noodles

Dust the chicken livers well with seasoned flour.

Heat the oil in a pan or wok and gently fry the bacon for 2–3
minutes. Remove to an ovenproof dish and add the green pepper and mushrooms to the pan. Lightly fry for 2 minutes, then
add the liver, tomatoes and herbs. Cook for a further 2 minutes.

Season to taste and transfer to the dish with the bacon. Cover
and bake for 25–30 minutes at 180°C/350°F/Gas Mark 4.

Cook the noodles as directed and serve with the liver.

Mexican bean stew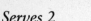

Serves 2

225 g/8 oz minced beef
1 tbsp sunflower oil
115 g/4 oz red/green/yellow peppers, chopped
1 clove garlic, crushed
1 tsp dried chives
small tin red kidney beans
small tin haricot or butter beans
small tin chopped tomatoes
chilli powder to taste
225 g/8 oz stock (see page 143)

Heat the oil in a pan or wok. Fry the beef, garlic and peppers for 5–6 minutes. Add the chives, beans, tomatoes and chilli powder.

Bring to the boil, then simmer for 15–20 minutes. Serve with rice.

All-in-one lamb hotpot

Serves 2

2 frozen lamb chops, thawed
little sunflower oil
1 large carrot, sliced
1 medium leek, sliced
a few frozen peas, thawed
115g (4 oz) cabbage chopped
1 clove garlic, very finely chopped
a sprig of rosemary
1 tbsp chopped parsley
450 ml/3/4 pint stock (see page 143)
medium sweet potato very finely sliced

Brown the lamb chops on both sides in a non-stick frying pan, then remove from the heat. Mix together all the prepared vegetables.

Place half the vegetable mixture in the bottom of an ovenproof dish, and put the chops on top. Lay the remaining vegetables over the chops.

Stir the garlic, rosemary and parsley into the stock and pour it into the pot. Cover with a layer of sweet potato and brush with oil. Cover and bake at 180°C/350°F/Gas Mark 4 for 25–30 minutes. Remove the lid and continue cooking, uncovered, for 30 minutes, or until the top is browned.

Pan-fried chicken livers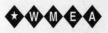

Serves 2

225 g/8 oz chicken livers
little gram flour for dusting
1 tbsp sunflower oil
1/2 tsp fresh chopped thyme
225 g/8 oz chicken stock (see page 143)
2 tbsp soya cream
1 tsp chives, chopped

Wash and prepare the chicken livers, pat them dry and dust over with the gram flour. Heat the oil in a shallow pan, add the liver and thyme and cook over moderate heat for 1 minute to seal.

Remove the liver, add the stock and bring it to the boil. Boil for 1 minute, scraping up the pieces from the pan. Reduce the heat, return the liver to the pan and poach over a gentle heat for 3–4 minutes, or until the liver is just cooked but a little pink in the middle. Lift out the meat and place on a warm plate. Add the cream to the stock and stir well.

Spoon the sauce over the liver and sprinkle with chives. Serve with either rice or noodles.

Bacon and potato scramble

Serves 2

1 large sweet potato, scrubbed
few small broad beans (fresh or frozen)
4 tbsp sunflower oil (preferably 'buttery' variety)
340 g/12 oz bacon pieces
2 small courgettes, thinly sliced
2 tomatoes, skinned, seeded and chopped into 25 mm/
   1 in pieces
1 tbsp chives, chopped
1 tbsp parsley, chopped
salt and pepper

Dressing: (omit for exclusion diet)
1 tbsp apple juice or rice vinegar
1 tsp honey
1 tsp wheat-free Dijon mustard

Cook the sweet potato in boiling salted water for about 8 minutes. Drain and cut into cubes. Boil the beans for approximately 6 minutes (they can be boiled with the sweet potato).

Heat the oil in a large size pan or wok, add the bacon pieces and chives and cook over a moderate heat for 3–4 minutes.

Remove the bacon from the pan, add the beans and courgettes and cook for 3–4 minutes. Add the sweet potato and tomatoes and continue cooking for 4–5 minutes, or until the vegetables are hot and cooked. Season to taste.

Return the bacon to the pan. Mix together all the ingredients for the dressing. Drizzle slowly over the scramble and sprinkle with parsley.

Baked porky pieces

Serves 2

225–280 g/8–10 oz pork stir fry
1 tbsp sunflower oil
1 tbsp fresh chives, chopped
1 tsp fresh thyme
1 clove garlic, crushed (optional)
115 g/4 oz mushrooms, chopped
225 g/8 oz chopped fresh tomatoes or drained, tinned tomatoes and 1 tbsp juice
salt and pepper

Heat the oil in a shallow pan and add the chives, thyme and garlic (if using). Fry for about 2 minutes over a gentle heat.

Add the pork pieces and seal, turning once. Transfer to an ovenproof dish along with the mushrooms. Pour over the tomatoes and season well.

Cover and bake for 40–45 minutes at 180°C/350°F/Gas Mark 4, and then bake uncovered for a further 10 minutes. Serve on a bed of rice noodles.

Coley courgette casserole

Serves 2

340 g/12 oz coley fillet, skinned
30 g/1 oz sunflower oil (preferably 'buttery' variety)
170 g/6 oz courgettes, thinly sliced
225 ml/8 fl oz fish stock (see page 143)
1½ tsp fresh mixed herbs (or ½ tsp dried herbs)
bouquet garni
1 tbsp arrowroot to thicken
2 tbsp frozen peas
2 large tomatoes, sliced
1 tsp paprika
salt and fresh ground black pepper

Cut the coley into 5 cm/2 in pieces. Heat the oil in a pan, add the courgettes and cook over a moderate heat for 2–3 minutes. Remove the courgettes from the pan and add the stock, herbs and bouquet garni. Bring to the boil and thicken with arrowroot.

Place the courgettes, fish, peas and tomato slices in an ovenproof dish, season with salt, pepper and paprika and pour over the thickened stock. Bake for 25–30 minutes at 180°C/350°F/Gas Mark 4, or until the fish is just cooked through.

Serve with rice noodles.

Spaghetti with vegetable sauce ◆ W M E

Serves 2

rice spaghetti (enough for two)
approximately 450 g/1 lb vegetables (e.g. leeks, carrots,
    swede, parsnips, celery)
300 ml/1/2 pint vegetable stock (see page 144)
1 bay-leaf
3 or 4 peppercorns
pinch nutmeg
salt and pepper
chopped parsley (optional)

Prepare the vegetables and chop fairly small. Bring the stock to the boil and add the vegetables, peppercorns, bay-leaf, salt and pepper. Cook gently for 30–40 minutes, or until the vegetables are soft. Add more water if necessary.

Remove from the heat and transfer to a blender. Process until more or less smooth. Return to the pan. (A little arrowroot can be added to thicken the sauce if necessary.) Stir in the nutmeg and leave to rest.

Cook the spaghetti for the required amount of time. During

the last few minutes reheat the sauce. Drain the spaghetti, put on a warmed plate and pour over the vegetable sauce. Sprinkle with parsley if using.

The sauce can be made the day before and stored in the refrigerator.

Vegetable rice

Serves 2

340 g/12 oz long-grain rice, cooked
60 g/2 oz sunflower oil (preferably 'buttery' variety)
1 orange or yellow pepper, seeded, cored and chopped
2 sticks celery, finely chopped
115 g/4 oz broccoli, chopped
2 large tomatoes, skinned, seeded and chopped
60–115 g/2–4 oz mushrooms, finely chopped
$1/4$ tsp cayenne pepper
salt
1 tbsp fresh chives, finely chopped

Heat the oil in a large pan. Add the celery, pepper and broccoli. Stir fry for 8–10 minutes, or until the vegetables are softened. Add the tomatoes and mushrooms. Continue cooking for a further 5–6 minutes, stirring frequently.

Add salt to taste and the cayenne pepper. Stir in the rice and combine all the ingredients. Continue stirring over the heat for 8–10 minutes, or until thoroughly heated through. Remove from the heat, stir in the chopped chives and serve.

SOUPS AND STARTERS

Gamekeeper's pot ◆ⓌⓂⒺ

Serves 4

1 medium leek
1 large carrot
1 small celery stick
1 small parsnip
1 piece of swede
850 ml/1½ pints chicken stock (see page 143)
60 g/2 oz lean bacon pieces, finely chopped and soaked free
    of salt
1 tbsp cooked lentils
sprig of parsley
small piece bay-leaf
1 sage leaf
pinch dried thyme
salt and pepper

Wash and prepare the vegetables, chopping them into small pieces.

Put them in a large saucepan with the bacon, lentils, herbs and seasoning to taste.

Cover and simmer for 1 hour. Remove the bay-leaf, set aside to cool, then liquidize to a coarse texture.

Cream of carrot soup ◆ⓌⓂⒺ

Serves 4

450 g/1 lb carrots, washed, peeled and chopped
1 stick celery, chopped
115 g/4 oz swede, chopped
60 g/2 oz lean unsmoked bacon, chopped
2 good spikes chives, chopped
850 ml/1½ pints chicken stock (see page 143)
30 g/1 oz dairy-free margarine

2 tbsp arrowroot
bouquet garni
salt and pepper
little soya cream or creamed coconut*
chopped parsley to garnish

Lightly fry the vegetables for 3–4 minutes in the margarine; do not allow them to colour. Add chopped bacon and chives and continue to fry for another 2–3 minutes.

Add the stock, bouquet garni and seasoning and simmer for 3/4–1 hour or until the vegetables are soft. Remove the bouquet garni and liquidize. Return to the pan and adjust seasoning if necessary.

Blend the arrowroot with a little water, add a little of the hot soup and mix well. Add to the contents in the pan and heat to thicken, stirring, for 2 minutes.

When ready to serve, reheat gently and swirl in the cream to the required consistency. Sprinkle with chopped parsley.

* If creamed coconut is used, reduce the amount of salt added.

Asparagus soup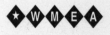

Serves 4

1 large bundle fresh or frozen asparagus
2 sticks celery
600 ml/1 pint chicken stock (see page 143)
parsley, chopped (to taste)
chives, finely chopped (to taste)
2 tbsp light olive oil or sunflower oil
salt and pepper

Chop the celery into small pieces. In a roomy pan, heat the olive oil, add the celery and chives and cook until the celery begins to soften.

Add the asparagus and stir round for 2 minutes. Pour in the stock to almost cover, add the parsley and season to taste.

Bring to the boil, then reduce the heat to a low simmer for about 30 minutes, or until the asparagus is soft.

Remove from the heat, leave to cool and then liquidize until smooth. When required, return to the pan and heat gently.

Mushroom soup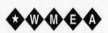

Serves 3

1 medium spike chives
400 g/14 oz mushrooms
300 ml/¹/₂ pint chicken or vegetable stock (see page 143)
¹/₄ tsp oregano
170 g/6 oz soya cream mixed with 115 g/4 oz cold water
arrowroot to thicken
chopped parsley to garnish

Wash and slice the mushrooms. Put them in a saucepan with the stock, chive and oregano. Simmer for 20 minutes.

Remove from the heat and allow to cool a little. Add the soya cream and water mixture and stir well.

Liquidize the mushroom and stock mixture, return to the heat and thicken with a little arrowroot.

Add the cream mixture, pour into bowls and sprinkle with chopped parsley.

Cream of watercress

Serves 3

225 g/8 oz packet watercress
1 medium stick celery, finely chopped
1 dessertspoon sunflower oil
600 ml/1 pint chicken stock (see page 143)
1 dessertspoon arrowroot
salt and pepper
1 dessertspoon soya cream
chopped parsley to garnish

Wash the watercress well and check for tough stalks. Gently heat the oil in a pan and sweat the watercress for 2 minutes. Remove the watercress, put the celery in the pan and cook until soft. Return the watercress to the pan, add the stock and season to taste. Simmer gently for 8–10 minutes.

Mix the arrowroot with a little water, add 1 tbsp soup, mix well and liquidize until smooth.

Return to the pan and reheat very gently, taking care not to allow the soup to boil. When ready to serve, swirl in a dessert-spoon of soya cream and sprinkle with chopped parsley.

A sort of boullabaise

Serves 4

225–280 g/8–10 oz white fish fillet
600 ml/1 pint fish stock (see page 143) or water, or water
    and white wine (if allowed)
1 small to medium carrot
1 stick celery
8 cm/3 in leek
1 very small turnip
1 small tin tomatoes
1 heaped tsp tomato purée
1 small garlic clove, crushed
bouquet garni
sprig fresh dill, chopped
salt and pepper
parsley to garnish

Wash and skin the fish and remove any obvious bones. Wash and finely chop all the vegetables.

Put the vegetables and garlic in a saucepan, lay the fish on top and add the stock, tomatoes, purée, herbs (except the parsley) and seasoning. Bring to the boil and simmer for 30 minutes. Remove the bouquet garni and check seasoning.

Serve in individual bowls; the fish will break into pieces naturally. Sprinkle well with parsley.

Chilled cucumber soup   ◆ⓌⓂⒺⒶ

Serves 4

2 spikes chives, finely chopped
1 large cucumber, peeled and finely chopped
2 small to medium sprigs mint
750 ml/1¼ pint vegetable or chicken stock (see page 143)
1 level tbsp arrowroot
salt and pepper
little soya cream
green pure food colouring (optional)

Place the chives, cucumber, mint, stock and seasoning in a saucepan. Simmer gently for 25–30 minutes or until the cucumber is soft. Transfer to a liquidizer or blender and process until smooth.

Mix the arrowroot with a little cold water to a cream, add a little hot soup, mix well and return to the pan. Reheat gently, stirring, until the soup has thickened. Continue to cook, stirring, for a further 1–2 minutes.

Remove from the heat, allow to cool a little, stir in the soya cream and test the seasoning. If required, 1–2 drops of green pure food colouring can be added. Pour into a suitable sized bowl or tureen and chill.

For dinner parties, this soup can be served sprinkled with a mixture of finely diced cucumber, mint leaves and small green grape halves.

Lentil soup   ◆ⓌⓂⒺ

Serves 4

170 g/6 oz lentils
2 rashers streaky unsmoked bacon, finely chopped
2 spikes chives
1 small stick celery, chopped
1 small carrot, chopped
2 plum tomatoes, skinned and chopped
850–1150 ml/1½–2 pints chicken stock (see page 143)
bouquet garni
small knob dairy-free margarine
parsley to garnish

Put all the ingredients except the margarine and parsley in a pan. Bring to the boil and simmer for 1½–1¾ hours.

Remove the bouquet garni, transfer to a blender and liquidize. Return to the pan and reheat, briskly stirring in the margarine.

Serve sprinkled with plenty of fresh chopped parsley.

Cream of tomato soup

Serves 4

675 g/1½ lb tomatoes, washed, quartered and seeds
    removed
1 tbsp sunflower oil
1 small stick celery, chopped
1 carrot chopped
30–60 g/1–2 oz lean unsmoked bacon
2 spikes chives, chopped
600 ml/1 pint chicken stock (see page 143)
2 tsp tomato purée
1½ tbsp arrowroot
bouquet garni
4–6 peppercorns, depending on taste
1 tsp demerara sugar
salt
little soya cream
chopped basil leaves to garnish

Lightly fry the celery, carrot, bacon and chives in the oil for 3–4 minutes or until soft but not coloured. Add the tomatoes, stock, purée, bouquet garni and peppercorns. Cover and simmer for 25–30 minutes or until the vegetables are soft. Remove the bouquet garni and liquidize. Return to the pan. Add the sugar and season to taste with salt.

Mix the arrowroot with a little water to a cream consistency, add a little hot soup, mix well and return to pan. Bring to boil and stir for 2 minutes. Allow to cool slightly, then swirl in the amount of cream required and sprinkle generously with fresh torn basil leaves.

Cream of cauliflower soup   ◆★◆W◆M◆E◆A◆

Serves 4

1 fresh white cauliflower
1 tbsp sunflower oil
600–750 ml/1–1¼ pints chicken or vegetable stock (see
    pages 143–4)
1-2 level tbsp arrowroot
salt and pepper
good pinch grated nutmeg
little soya cream
chopped parsley to garnish

Break up the cauliflower into sprigs, discard the green leaves
and wash well in salted water.

Heat the oil and stock in a pan. Mix the arrowroot with
a little water, add a little hot stock, mix well and return to
the pan. Season to taste. The mixture should have a creamy
consistency. Add the cauliflower and grated nutmeg.

Cover and simmer for 20–35 minutes or until the cauliflower is well cooked. Liquidize soup and reheat gently. Swirl
in the cream and sprinkle with chopped parsley.

Harvest vegetable soup   ◆★◆W◆M◆E◆A◆

Serves 2–3

450 g/1 lb root vegetables (e.g. carrots, swede, turnip, leeks,
    parsnips, celery, celeriac, sweet potato)
stock, preferably beef (if not, chicken or vegetable – see
    pages 143–4)
6 peppercorns
good pinch grated nutmeg
1 bay-leaf
bouquet garni

Cut the vegetables into smallish pieces and put in a roomy
pan. Almost cover with stock, then add the peppercorns, bay-
leaf, nutmeg and bouquet garni.

Bring to the boil, skim off any scum then lower the heat to

a simmer. Simmer for 3/4 hour. Check that the vegetables are soft, remove the peppercorns and bay-leaf and leave to cool.

When cool, blend the soup to a coarse consistency. Adjust the seasoning and add a further pinch of nutmeg if needed.

Reheat when needed. This soup keeps well in the refrigerator for 2–3 days. It also freezes well.

Mushrooms in garlic sauce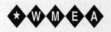

Serves 2

340 g/12 oz mushrooms, cut into chunks
2 or 3 cloves garlic (depending on size), crushed
225–280 g/8–10 oz chicken stock (see page 143)
2 tbsp sunflower oil (preferably 'buttery' variety)
1/3 tsp dried oregano
salt and pepper
little arrowroot

Put the oil in a medium-sized pan and heat. Add the mushrooms and garlic and sauté for 3–4 minutes over a medium to high heat.

Add 225 g/8 oz stock and the oregano, reduce the heat and simmer for about 8–10 minutes or until the mushrooms are cooked. Add the extra stock if necessary. Season to taste.

Remove from the heat. Add a little arrowroot to some cold water and mix with a little stock. Stir into the sauce to thicken to a creamy consistency.

Serve with rice cakes.

Tropical ham salad

Serves 1

1 piece mango and pineapple chopped
60 g/2 oz lean ham, chopped
portion of lettuce
salt and black pepper
few drops pineapple juice
toasted pine nuts or toasted sunflower seeds to garnish

Wash and dry the lettuce leaves. Season the pineapple juice with a few grains of salt and some pepper. Lightly sprinkle this over lettuce leaves and line a dish with them.

Mix the chopped fruit and ham together and place on the lettuce. Sprinkle with pine nuts or sunflower seeds.

Potted ham   W M E

Serves 4

225 g/8 oz cooked ham, finely chopped
85 g/3 oz sunflower oil
1/2 tsp wheat-free Dijon mustard
1 tbsp chopped parsley
salt and pepper
little dairy-free margarine, melted

Put the first four ingredients in a blender and process until smooth. Season to taste.

Remove and put in a suitable clean dish. Cover with melted margarine and refrigerate.

This mixture can be put in individual pots and used as a starter. It is also very good for packed lunches.

Weekday tuna pâté   ★ W M E

Serves 2

200g/7 oz tin tuna in spring water
2 heaped tsp tomato purée
small knob dairy-free margarine
1–2 drops pure basil oil or 1 tbsp fresh basil leaves, chopped

Drain the tuna well and put it in a blender. Add the other ingredients and blend until well mixed and smooth. Put in a suitable ceramic dish, cover with cling film and chill well.

It is not necessary to use additional margarine when spreading this pâté.

Sunday salmon pâté

Serves 2

1 salmon fillet
6 peppercorns
good sprig parsley
good sprig dill, finely chopped
little fish stock (see page 143)
knob dairy-free margarine
3–4 drops rice vinegar

Place the salmon in an ovenproof dish, add the peppercorns
and parsley and pour over a little fish stock. Cover with a lid
or foil and poach in the oven at 180°C/350°F/Gas Mark 4
until just cooked through.

Remove from the oven and leave to cool in poaching
liquid. When cold, remove the skin from the salmon and place
it in a blender with the chopped dill, margarine and rice
vinegar. Blend until well mixed. Transfer to a ceramic dish,
cover with cling film and chill well.

Dinner party starter

Serves 2

Sunday salmon pâté (see above)
small asparagus tips (4 per person)
few cucumber slices and mint leaves, to garnish

Vinaigrette dressing:
1 tsp wheat-free Dijon mustard
1 tbsp rice vinegar
1/4 tsp salt and black pepper
1/2 tsp sugar
2 tbsp light olive oil

Put all the ingredients for the vinaigrette into a blender or
screw-top jar, blend together and store in the refrigerator.
Shake before use. (Any left-over vinaigrette can be kept in the
refrigerator for up to 5 days.)

Line a small oblong tin or individual ramekin dishes with cling film. Two-thirds fill with salmon pâté and leave to chill.

Steam the asparagus for 3–4 minutes, keeping it slightly crunchy. Remove from the heat and drain. Turn out the pâté and place a slice on each plate (or turn out each ramekin onto a plate). Lightly dip each asparagus spear in the vinaigrette. Arrange 4 on each plate in a lattice pattern around the fish.

Decorate the salmon with cucumber slices and mint leaves.

Baked stuffed tomatoes

Serves 2

4 firm medium tomatoes
2 heaped tbsp brown rice, cooked
1 tbsp chopped green pepper
1 tbsp grated celeriac or finely chopped celery
1 tbsp mushrooms, finely chopped
1 dessertspoon parsley, chopped
1 heaped tsp fresh thyme
salt and pepper
small knob dairy-free margarine
oil for brushing

Wash the tomatoes, cut off the tops for lids and scoop out the seeds.

Mix together the rice, pepper, celeriac, mushrooms and herbs. Season to taste. Pile the mixture into the tomato cases, put a tiny knob of margarine on top of the filling and put on the lid.

Stand the tomatoes in a square or rectangular dish, brush them lightly with oil and cover with a lid or tin foil.

Bake in a preheated oven at 200°C/400°F/Gas Mark 6 for 15 minutes. Then remove the lid or foil and continue baking for about 8 minutes, or until the tomatoes are crisp but not wrinkled.

Serve with a salad garnish. If served with a full salad and crispy bread, this makes an ideal supper dish.

Sautéed scallops   ◆W◆M◆E◆A

Serves 2

8–10 large scallops
a few drops rice vinegar
1 tbsp flour
salt and pepper
1 tbsp light olive oil mixed with 30g/1oz dairy-free margarine
watercress and cucumber to garnish

Trim the scallops (or get the fishmonger to do it for you when
you buy them. Wash them well and dry them on kitchen paper.

Very lightly sprinkle the scallops with rice vinegar, season
to taste, then toss them in gram flour.

Heat a large pan, add the oil and margarine and drop in the
scallops; do not overcrowd them. Sauté until golden, turning
once, for about 8–10 minutes. Transfer to a warmed dish and
serve garnished with watercress leaves and cucumber slices.

FISH

Baked trout with cucumber sauce   ◆W◆M◆E◆A

Serves 2

2 trout, cleaned
2 small bay-leaves
30 g/1 oz dairy-free margarine, melted
2 sprigs dill
salt and pepper
1 medium cucumber
little olive oil
little white grape juice or apple juice

Wash and dry the trout, removing the head and tail if wished.
Sprinkle the inside of the trout with salt and pepper and place
the bay-leaf and dill inside. Brush inside and out with melted
margarine.

Wrap the fish in foil and bake at 180°C/350°F/Gas Mark 4 for approximately 20 minutes.

Meanwhile, peel the cucumber and cut it into small chunks. Heat the oil in a shallow pan, add the cucumber and sauté over a gentle heat until soft. Remove from the heat and take out 1 tbsp cucumber with a slotted spoon. Transfer the remaining cucumber to blender and process until smooth, adding 1–2 tbsp grape or apple juice to reach the required consistency.

Add a pinch of salt and the reserved cucumber, mix together and serve with the baked trout. May be served hot or cold.

Stuffed cod steaks with watercress sauce   ◆ W M E A

Serves 2

2 cod steaks
2 tsp multi-coloured peppercorns, crushed
1–2 tbsp olive oil
salt and pepper
170 g/6 oz watercress
small knob dairy-free margarine
salt
pinch nutmeg
1–2 tbsp chicken stock (see page 143)

Heat the oil in a pan, wipe the cod steaks and brush with oil. Press the crushed peppercorns onto both sides of the steaks. (You can sprinkle the crushed peppercorns on and gently roll a rolling pin over for the steaks to stick them on firmly). Season and place in the pan. Cook over a low heat until the fish are cooked, turning once.

Meanwhile, remove the coarse stalks from the watercress and wash well. Heat the margarine in a pan, add the watercress, nutmeg and sweat, stirring continuously, until wilted.

Transfer to a blender and process on the pulse switch to avoid over-processing. Add chicken stock to reach the required consistency.

This dish is ideal served with baked sweet potato, carrot and leek batons.

Tuna quickie

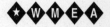

Serves 2

200g/7oz tin tuna in spring water
$^1/_2$–1 tsp wheat-free korma curry powder (check ingredients
   carefully)
2 tsp olive oil
$^1/_4$–$^1/_2$ tsp paprika
small tub soya yoghurt

Grease an ovenproof dish, drain the tuna and place in the dish. Add the spices to the oil and mix well. Stir in the yoghurt.

Spread the mixture over the tuna, cover and bake for 15–20 minutes at 180°C/350°F/Gas Mark 4 until heated through.

Serve with saffron rice and steamed asparagus.

Plaice and celery parcels

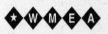

Serves 2

2 plaice double fillets, skinned
2 celery sticks, cut into thin matchsticks
1 carrot, cut into thin matchsticks
1 courgette, cut into thin matchsticks
115 g/4 oz chestnut mushrooms, wiped and thinly sliced
fresh parsley
celery salt and pepper to taste
2 tbsp vegetable or fish stock (see page 143)

Heat the oven to 180°C/350°F/Gas Mark 4. Prepare 2 double sheets of buttered foil. Place the celery, carrot and courgette matchsticks in portions on the 2 pieces of foil and season lightly.

Put a portion of mushrooms on one half of each plaice fillet and roll it up. Place on top of the vegetables. Season the plaice and lay a sprig of parsley on top. Pour over 1 tbsp stock.

Wrap the foil over the fish to enclose completely.

Place in a baking dish and bake for about 20 minutes or until the fish is tender.

Seafood with noodles

Serves 2

280 g/10 oz seafood salad or mixture of prawns, scallops
    and mussels
1–2 tbsp sunflower or olive oil
1 medium carrot, cut into batons
1 medium stick celery, cut into batons
1/2 green pepper, cut into fine strips
few pieces fresh pineapple or mango
good pinch ground ginger
small amount of water chestnuts (if available)
1 tbsp fresh chopped coriander
1–2 tbsp apple juice
good pinch paprika
rice noodles

Cook the rice noodles as required and keep warm.

Heat the oil in a pan, add the ginger and stir well. Add the carrot and celery batons and sauté for 5–6 minutes, add the courgette and pepper, then cook for a further 3–4 minutes. Add the seafood, pineapple or mango, water chestnuts if using, coriander and apple juice. Stir well and poach over gentle heat for 3–4 minutes.

Pour freshly boiled water through the rice noodles to reheat, drain and place on a warm serving plate. Spoon the seafood mixture over the noodles and sprinkle with paprika.

Seafood pasta salad

Serves 2

225–280 g/8–10 oz seafood salad
2 spikes chives, chopped
170 g/6 oz mushrooms, sliced
280–340 g/10–12 oz chopped tomatoes, tinned or bottled
1 dessertspoon sundried tomato paste
1/2 tsp powdered garlic
1/4 tsp thyme, chopped
1 tsp basil leaves, torn into pieces
1 tbsp sunflower or olive oil
salt and pepper
2 servings rice pasta, cooked as required

Heat the oil in a pan and add the chives and mushrooms. Cook for 3–4 minutes over a moderate heat. Add the tomatoes, tomato paste, garlic, thyme and basil and season to taste.

Cook over a gentle heat for 6–8 minutes, add the seafood salad and poach in the tomato and mushroom sauce over a low heat for 3–4 minutes.

Pour boiling water through the pasta to reheat, shake well and transfer to serving dish. Pour the seafood and sauce over the pasta and sprinkle with parsley if desired. A bowl of green salad will complement this dish well.

Plaice turbans in mushroom sauce

Serves 2

4 medium plaice fillets
salt and black pepper
350 g/12 oz mushrooms, thinly sliced
225 ml/8 fl oz fish or vegetable stock (see page 143)
115–140 g/4–5 oz soya cream
pinch oregano
fresh parsley, chopped, to garnish

Wash and dry the plaice fillets, season lightly and roll up. Secure them with a cocktail stick if necessary. Transfer to suitable ovenproof dish.

Put the stock, mushrooms and oregano in a saucepan. Simmer for 6–8 minutes, until mushrooms are tender. Pour over the plaice, cover and bake at 180°C/350°F/Gas Mark 4 for 10–12 minutes, or until the fish is just cooked through. Remove from the oven, drain the liquid from the fish and transfer to a pan. Cover and keep warm.

Boil the liquid to reduce by about a third, then add the cream. Check the seasoning, stir well to mix and pour over the fish. Sprinkle generously with parsley.

Baked mackerel with gooseberry sauce

Serves 2

2 medium mackerel, cleaned and filleted
1 tsp rice vinegar
1 small knob dairy-free margarine
$1/2$ tsp dried mixed herbs
salt and pepper
225 g/8 oz gooseberries, topped and tailed
1–2 tbsp caster sugar
30 g/1 oz dairy-free margarine
115 ml/4 fl oz water

Wash and dry the mackerel fillets, place in an ovenproof dish and sprinkle the dried herbs on top. Season lightly, add a knob of margarine and pour over a little water and rice vinegar. Cover and bake at 180°C/350°F/Gas Mark 4 for 15–20 minutes, or until fish flakes are soft to the touch.

Meanwhile, wash the gooseberries, place them in a pan with the sugar and water and cook until the gooseberries have popped open and are beginning to blend (about 5 minutes). Remove from heat and beat in the margarine.

Pour a spoonful of the gooseberry sauce over the mackerel

fillets. Serve the rest of the sauce in a sauce boat. Wild rice and a salsa of choice go well with this dish.

POULTRY

Chicken and apple bake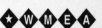

Serves 2

1 tbsp sunflower oil
340 g/12 oz chicken, cut into cubes
2 spikes chives, finely chopped
1 large stick celery, sliced
2 medium sweet potatoes
3 or 4 stems fresh thyme
1 medium cooking apple
1 small bay-leaf
30 g/1 oz Puy lentils
300 ml/¹/₂ pint chicken stock (see page 143)

Heat the oil in a medium frying pan, add the chicken and fry for 3–4 minutes, until lightly browned. Transfer to a casserole.

Put the celery in the pan, cook for 3–4 minutes, then add to the casserole. Peel, core and finely chop the apple, and add to the casserole with the chopped chives, thyme and bay-leaf. Add the lentils and stock. Stir well to mix. Cover and cook at 180°C/350°F/Gas Mark 4 for about an hour, or until the meat and lentils are cooked.

Remove from the oven and stir well for the cooked apple to thicken the sauce. (If it is not thick enough add a little arrowroot mixed in water and return to the oven until the sauce thickens.)

Steam the sweet potatoes until just tender, cool and rinse under cold water. Slice very thinly and layer over the dish. Brush with oil and put under a heated grill until the potatoes are lightly browned.

If preferred, the sweet potato topping can be omitted and the casserole served with boiled rice.

Westcountry chicken

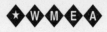

Serves 4

enough chicken drumsticks for 4 portions
300 ml/¹/₂ pint apple juice or white grape juice and 1 tsp
   caster sugar (omit sugar for arthritis exclusion diet)
medium sprig fresh rosemary
2 or 3 mint leaves
1 tbsp gram flour
1 tbsp light olive oil
salt and pepper
1 tbsp sweet red pepper, chopped
2 small courgettes, cut into rings
¹/₄ tsp ground garlic
1 tbsp white wine (optional)
little oil for frying

Mix the apple or grape juice with the oil and season.

Place the drumsticks in a shallow glass or ceramic dish, tuck the herbs around them and pour over the marinade. Leave in the refrigerator overnight.

Remove the chicken from the marinade and drain. Toss in gram flour. Heat a little oil in a pan, fry the chicken until lightly golden and transfer to an ovenproof dish. Add the peppers and courgettes. Stir the ground garlic into the marinade and white wine if using. Pour over the chicken and bake at 180°C/350°F/Gas Mark 4 for 25–30 minutes.

Remove the chicken from the oven and keep warm. Boil the liquid until reduced by one-third, check the seasoning and thicken with a little arrowroot if desired.

Serve on a bed of rice noodles.

Chicken fricassée

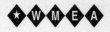

4 generous servings

4 good-sized chicken portions or required quantity of chicken
   stir-fry pieces
340 ml/12 fl oz chicken stock (see page 143)
1/2 sweet red pepper, chopped
few fine green beans, chopped
few broad beans, chopped
few asparagus spears, chopped
60 g/2 oz dairy-free margarine, melted
60 g/2 oz flour mix (see page 158) or arrowroot
170 ml/6 fl oz soya milk
3–4 tbsp soya cream
salt and pepper
chopped parsley to garnish

Wipe the chicken portions clean, place them in an ovenproof
dish, cover with stock and bake at 180°C/350°F/Gas Mark 4
for approximately 3/4 hour, or until the chicken is tender and
cooked through. Remove from the oven, cool, then remove
the flesh from the bones.

Steam the chopped vegetables and keep warm.

In a saucepan, combine the margarine, flour, milk and
170 g/6 oz chicken stock. Whisk over a medium heat until
the sauce boils and thickens. Add the chicken, vegetables and
seasoning. Reheat and stir in the cream.

Sprinkle with parsley and serve with a bowl of rice. The
extra chicken stock can be saved, refrigerated and used next
day or put into ice-cube tray, frozen and used later.

Curried chicken goujons   ◆W◆M◆E

Serves 2

2 chicken breasts
2 or 3 medium spikes chives, very finely chopped
2 small cloves garlic, crushed
2 tsp wheat-free korma curry powder (check ingredients
     carefully)
1/2 tsp salt
good pinch cayenne pepper
1 heaped tbsp tomato purée
2 tbsp sunflower oil
gram flour to coat
parsley to garnish

Skin the chicken and remove any bones. Cut into thick finger
lengths.

Stir the chives, garlic, curry powder, salt and cayenne
pepper into the tomato purée. Brush this mixture all over the
goujons, cover and chill for 1¹/₂–2 hours.

Heat the oil in a pan or wok. Coat the chicken on all sides
with gram flour, place in pan and cook on a moderate heat for
6–8 minutes until lightly crisp. Serve garnished with chopped
parsley.

Chicken in tarragon cream   ◆W◆M◆E◆A

Serves 2

2 chicken breasts
1 tbsp chopped leek
1–2 tbsp sunflower oil
1 clove garlic, crushed
1 tbsp fresh tarragon
85 g/3 oz mushrooms, finely sliced
225–280 ml/8–10 fl oz chicken stock (see page 143)
115 g/4 oz soya cream
salt and pepper

Heat 1 tbsp oil in a pan or wok. Remove the skin and cut the chicken into cubes. Sauté in the pan for a few minutes until lightly browned. Remove and drain on kitchen paper.

Add a little more oil to the pan if necessary, and fry the leek and garlic and until the leek is softened but not browned. Add the mushroom slices and cook for a further 3–4 minutes.

Return the chicken to the pan with the stock and tarragon and poach gently until the chicken is tender. Remove from the heat, season to taste and stir in the cream. Return to the heat for 1–2 minutes, until thoroughly reheated.

Serve with rice or noodles.

Chicken risotto

Serves 2

225–280 g/8–10 oz chicken, cooked and chopped
1 tbsp sunflower oil
60 g/2 oz bacon pieces, chopped
1 small leek, chopped
1 stick celery, chopped
1 green pepper, de-seeded and chopped
85 g/3 oz red kidney beans, cooked
60 g/2 oz mushrooms, sliced
1 clove garlic, crushed
225 g/8 oz patna or basmati rice
450–600 ml/^{3}/4–1 pint chicken stock (see page 143)
1 tbsp mixed fresh herbs, e.g. marjoram, basil, thyme.

Heat the oil in a large pan, add the bacon and leeks and cook for 3–4 minutes. Add the other vegetables and cook for 2–3 minutes. Add the rice and stir until the rice is transparent.

Add just under half of the stock, and the garlic, herbs and seasoning. Cook over a moderate heat, stirring frequently. Continue to cook adding stock as necessary, until the rice is just cooked.

Add the chicken, stir well and cook until the liquid is absorbed.

Brittany chicken

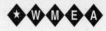

Serves 2

1 whole chicken breast
sunflower oil
1 tsp caraway seeds
300–450 ml/^{1}/2–^{3}/4 pint apple juice
1 sage leaf
2 courgettes, diagonally sliced
2 medium Cox's apples, cored but not peeled
little dairy-free margarine
toasted pine nuts (optional)

Open out the chicken breast and beat with a rolling pin until evenly flattened. Brush the inside surface with oil. Heat a frying pan, place the chicken breast in it and seal, turning until lightly golden.

Transfer to an ovenproof dish. Add sufficient apple juice to come half- to three-quarters of the way up the dish (the chicken does not need to be covered), and the sage leaf if using, and cook in the oven at 180°C/350°F/Gas Mark 4 for about ^{3}/4 hour. Twenty minutes before the end of the cooking time add the courgettes to the casserole.

Heat a clean frying pan and add a little sunflower oil and a knob of dairy-free margarine. Thickly slice the apples and add to the pan. Sauté until golden, turn and cook until other side is golden. Keep warm.

Remove the chicken from the casserole, cut into 2 cm/^{3}/4 in slices and lay on a plate. Remove the courgettes. Place on one side of the chicken, with the sautéed apple rings on the other. Toasted pine nuts can be sprinkled over if wished.

Chicken with grapes

Serves 4

4 chicken suprêmes
1 tbsp flour mix (see page 158 or use sago, tapioca or gram
  flour)
1 tbsp fresh sage, chopped
150 ml/5 fl oz white grape juice
40–60 g/1 1/2–2 oz dairy-free margarine
1/4 tsp vanilla essence
salt and pepper
handful seedless grapes
required amount of either rice pasta or rice noodles
small knob of dairy-free margarine
1 tbsp fresh basil leaves

Check the chicken to remove any skin or bones, wipe clean
and if necessary flatten to an even thickness.

Mix two-thirds of the sage with the flour and coat the
chicken pieces. Melt the margarine in a pan and add the
vanilla essence. Stir well. Add the chicken and cook over a
moderate heat until tender and lightly golden brown.

Remove from the pan and keep warm. Cook the pasta or
noodles, drain, rinse and drain. Stir in the margarine and
basil. Meanwhile, add the grape juice to the chicken pan and
mix with the remaining pan juices. Bring to the boil and
reduce by half. Add the grapes and continue cooking for
1–1 1/2 minutes. Pour over the chicken and serve.

Serve with roasted fennel and asparagus.

Turkey fusilli

Serves 4

675 g/1½ lb boneless turkey breast, cut into chunks
2 tbsp either rice or gram flour or flour mix (see page 158)
2 tbsp olive oil
1 clove garlic, crushed
½ green pepper, ½ red pepper and ½ yellow or orange
    pepper, each cored, de-seeded and sliced
225 g/8 oz chestnut mushrooms
1 medium courgette, sliced
400 g/14 oz tin or jar of chopped tomatoes
1 tsp oregano, dried
3 spikes chives, finely chopped
salt and pepper to taste
parsley to garnish

Coat the turkey in flour, then fry in the oil in a large pan until browned all over. Remove from the pan with a slotted spoon and set aside.

Fry the garlic, peppers, mushrooms and courgette in the oil remaining in the pan for 3–4 minutes. Add the passata, salt and pepper. Bring to the boil, lower the heat and return the turkey to pan. Simmer gently for 20 minutes, until turkey is cooked and tender.

Serve with rice pasta, well sprinkled with fresh parsley.

Crock-pot chicken casserole ◆ⓌⓂⒺ

Serves 4

4 chicken joints
1 medium leek, finely chopped
1 dessertspoon sunflower oil
600–850 ml/1–1½ pint chicken stock (see page 143)
2 tbsp tomato purée
bouquet garni
salt and pepper
arrowroot to thicken

Remove any skin from the chicken joints and lay in a crock pot or greased casserole.

Heat the oil in a pan and cook the leek until almost soft, remove with a slotted spoon and put in the casserole dish. Into same pan pour the stock, tomato purée and bouquet garni. Stir to combine the sediment from the leeks and bring to the boil. Thicken with arrowroot, season to taste and pour into the casserole.

Set the crock pot as directed or transfer to the oven and cook at 160°C/325°F/Gas Mark 3 for 1½–2 hours.

Chicken and sweet pepper casserole

Serves 4–6

900 g/2 lb chicken thighs
2–3 tbsp sunflower oil
340 g/12 oz mixed coloured peppers, de-seeded and
    chopped
170 g/6 oz mushrooms sliced
1 stick celery, chopped
1 tbsp gram flour
2 tsp paprika
2 tsp tomato purée
450–600 ml/¾–1 pint chicken stock (see page 143)
salt and pepper
parsley to garnish

Heat the oil in a pan or wok and fry the chicken until lightly browned. Transfer to a casserole. Add the peppers, mushrooms and celery to the pan and cook for 2–3 minutes. Transfer to the casserole with a slotted spoon.

Add the flour and paprika to the pan, stir well and cook for 1–2 minutes. Add the stock, purée and seasoning, scrape up the sediment from the chicken and vegetables and bring to the boil.

Pour into the casserole, transfer to the oven and cook for about 1 hour on 180°C/350°F/Gas Mark 4.

Serve sprinkled with parsley. This casserole goes well with any kind of rice.

BEEF

Braised steak with lentils   ◆W◆M◆E◆

Serves 4

4 pieces lean braising steak
170 g/6 oz mushrooms, sliced
2 sticks celery, chopped
170 g/6 oz red lentils, prepared
600 ml/1 pint good beef stock (see page 143)
4 tomatoes, skinned, seeded and cut into pieces
bouquet garni
salt and pepper
1 clove garlic, crushed
little arrowroot to thicken (optional)

Spread a mixture of half the mushrooms, celery and lentils over the base of an oblong ovenproof dish. Lay pieces of braising steak on the vegetables and add the tomatoes. Sprinkle with salt and pepper and add the bouquet garni.

Add the remaining mushrooms, celery and lentils and the garlic. Pour over the stock, cover and cook at 180°C/350°F/ Gas Mark 4 for 2–2½ hours.

Thicken with a little arrowroot if desired.

Steak pie   ◆W◆M◆E◆

Serves 4

450 g/1 lb lean braising steak, cubed
1 tbsp sunflower oil
1 large leek, finely chopped
225 g/8 oz mushrooms, sliced
600 ml/1 pint beef or vegetable stock (see page 143)

1 tbsp tomato purée
bouquet garni
1 bay-leaf
salt and pepper
little arrowroot to thicken
wheat-free shortcrust pastry using 170 g/6 oz flour mix (see
    page 158)
little soya milk

Heat oil in a frying pan, add the steak and cook until lightly browned. Transfer to a casserole. Fry the leek and mushrooms for 3–4 minutes and transfer to the casserole. Add the stock, tomato purée, bouquet garni and bay-leaf to the pan. Stir to de-glaze and season to taste.

Thicken with a little arrowroot and bring to boil, stirring. Simmer until the gravy thickens, for 2–3 minutes, pour into the casserole and cook at 180°C/350°F/Gas Mark 4 for 1½–2 hours.

Remove from the oven and discard the bay-leaf. Place the steak and vegetables in the base of a 1.5 l/2½ pint pie dish and spoon over 2–3 tablespoons of gravy, reserving the rest in a warm casserole.

Roll out the pastry and cut a 25 mm/1 in strip to go round the edge of the pie dish. Dampen the edge of the dish with water, place on the pastry strip and press down lightly. Dampen the top of the pastry strip with water. Place the rest of the pastry over the dish to form a lid and seal well round the edge. Cut two small slits on the lid, brush the top with soya milk and bake in a fairly hot oven until the pastry is cooked and golden.

Serve with the reserved gravy.

Goulash   W M E

Serves 4

450 g/1 lb lean stewing steak, cubed
1 tbsp oil
1 large leek, cut into rings
225 g/8 oz cabbage, shredded
2 tbsp tomato purée
170–225 ml/6–8 fl oz beef stock (see page 143)
2 tsp paprika
arrowroot to thicken
little soya cream
salt and pepper

Heat the oil in a medium-sized saucepan, add the steak and cook for 6–8 minutes to seal. Add the leek and cabbage and cook for a further 3–4 minutes.

Add the stock, purée and paprika and season to taste. Cover and simmer very gently for about an hour, or until meat is tender.

Remove from the heat and thicken with a little arrowroot to a creamy consistency. Stir in a little soya cream, check the seasoning and serve.

Rice noodles make an ideal accompaniment to this goulash.

Spaghetti bean bolognese   W M E

Serves 4

450 g/1 lb minced beef
115 g/4 oz bacon pieces, chopped
1 tbsp sunflower oil
1 stick celery, sliced
1 carrot, sliced
1 clove garlic, crushed
400g/14 oz tin or jar of chopped tomatoes

1 tbsp tomato purée
1/2 large tin mixed beans
1 tsp or cube wheat-free stock powder (check ingredients
   carefully)
2 tsp dried oregano
salt and pepper

Heat the oil in a saucepan and add the minced beef and bacon. Fry for 6 minutes, until beef is browned. Add the celery, carrot and garlic and cook for 3–4 minutes.

Add the remaining ingredients and simmer over a low heat for 30–40 minutes, then check the seasoning. Serve with spaghetti. This bean bolognese goes equally well with rice noodles.

LAMB

Lamb curry with pineapple and apricots

★ W M E

Serves 6

900 g/2 lb lean lamb, cubed
2 tbsp sunflower oil
170 g/6 oz leeks, cut into fine rings
2 tbsp gram flour
2 tbsp wheat-free korma curry powder (check ingredients
   carefully)
1 tsp ground ginger or 5 cm/2 in piece fresh ginger, grated
1 tsp ground coriander
340–400 g/12–14 oz chicken stock (see page 143)
225 g/8 oz creamed coconut
225 g/8 oz dried apricots
225 g/8 oz canned pineapple, drained
60 g/2 oz raisins

Heat the oil in a large pan, add the lamb and brown all over. Remove from the heat and keep warm. Add the leeks and cook until soft, without letting them brown.

Return the meat to the pan, sprinkle in the flour, ginger, curry powder and coriander and stir well. Add the stock and creamed coconut.

Bring to the boil, stir well and reduce to a simmer for 20 minutes. Add the apricots, pineapple and raisins, cover and simmer very gently for 1¼–1½ hours. Adjust seasoning and serve with rice.

Honey lamb

Serves 4

small to medium joint of lean lamb
Marinade:
170 ml/6 fl oz clear honey
2 small sprigs rosemary
170 ml/6 fl oz red grape juice
115–170 ml/4–6 fl oz concentrated pineapple juice
1 clove garlic, crushed

Mix together all the ingredients for the marinade. Place the lamb in a non-metallic bowl, pour over the marinade and leave in the refrigerator overnight.

Roast in the oven at 180°C/350°F/Gas Mark 4 for the required length of time (depending on weight of joint). Continue basting with the marinade during cooking.

Sweet and spicy lamb with rice

Serves 4

4 lamb steaks
1 tbsp sunflower oil
1 clove garlic, crushed

1 tin sliced peaches
1–2 tsp dried ginger (to taste)
2 tsp light brown or demerara sugar
pinch cumin
little arrowroot
white rice to serve 4
1 tbsp fresh thyme, chopped

Heat the oil in a pan, season the steaks, and add to the pan. Fry for 3–4 minutes, turning once, to lightly brown both sides. Remove the lamb from the pan.

Put the garlic, cumin, ginger and sugar and half the peach juice from the tin into the pan. Heat through, add a little arrowroot to thicken and bring to the boil. Lower the heat to a simmer, return the steaks to the sauce and leave on a low heat for 10–12 minutes.

Meanwhile, cook rice as required, drain and stir in the chopped thyme.

Remove the steaks and sauce from the heat, stir in the sliced peaches and serve with a portion of rice. An ideal accompaniment is steamed or roast asparagus.

Irish stew

Serves 4

8 middle neck lamb chops or scrag end of neck lamb
900 g/2 lb sweet potatoes, peeled and sliced
450 g/1 lb carrots, cut into small chunks
450 g/1 lb celery, cut into small pieces
1 tbsp chopped chives
salt and pepper
pinch mixed dried herbs
vegetable or chicken stock (see page 143)

Place half the lamb in the base of a casserole and add a sprinkling of chives. Then add half the carrot and celery followed by half the sweet potato. Repeat these layers, finishing with a layer of sweet potato.

Season the stock and pour into casserole to reach half-way up the side of the casserole. Sprinkle the herbs over the top.

Cover and cook at about 180°C/350°F/Gas Mark 4 for 2–3 hours.

Lamb kebabs

Serves 4

280 g/10 oz lean lamb, cubed
1 red pepper, de-seeded and cut into pieces
1 or 2 courgettes, cut into chunks
8 cherry tomatoes
8 button mushrooms

Marinade:
1 small tin vegetable juice
2 tsp wheat-free Worcestershire sauce (alternatively, use
    Mirrin – a sweet Japanese seasoning – or sweet rice
    vinegar, all available from good health-food shops)
salt and pepper
few fresh basil leaves, torn

Put the lamb in a non-metallic shallow dish. Mix the marinade ingredients together, pour over the lamb, cover and refrigerate overnight.

Remove the meat from the marinade. Blanch and drain the pepper and courgette pieces. Thread pieces of lamb, pepper, courgette, tomatoes and mushrooms alternately onto skewers.

Place the skewers across the grill pan, brush well with the marinade and grill for 20 minutes, turning and basting with the marinade.

Serve with saffron rice.

Lamb parcels

Serves 4

4 lamb chops, preferably lean and chump
4 large flat mushrooms
4 tomatoes, sliced
Heaped tsp dried mixed herbs
1 tbsp sunflower oil plus a little extra for brushing
salt and pepper

In a pan or wok, heat the oil and cook the chops to seal them
until they are lightly browned.

Remove them from the pan. Lay tomato slices on squares of
foil, season and sprinkle with herbs. Lay a chop on each base
of tomatoes, top with large flat mushrooms and brush with oil.

Fold the foil into parcels and bake at 180°C/350°F/Gas Mark
4 for 30–40 minutes, or until the chops are cooked and tender.

PORK

Cheat's chow mein

Serves 4

450 g/1 lb pork pieces
170 g/6 oz prawns
4 large chestnut mushrooms, cut into matchsticks
85–115 g/3–4 oz bean sprouts
small green pepper
2 large carrots, cut into batons
salt and black pepper
2 tbsp sunflower oil
300 ml/¹/₂ pint chicken stock (see page 143)
1 tsp Mirrin (Japanese sweet rice seasoning) or sweet rice
   vinegar available from good health food shops
rice noodles to serve 4

Cook the noodles as directed and keep warm.

Heat the oil in a pan or wok, add the carrots and green pepper and stir fry for 2–3 minutes. Add the pork and mushrooms and stir fry for 6–8 minutes. Add the bean sprouts and salt and pepper to taste and continue to stir fry for 1½–2 minutes.

Add the stock and Mirrin and cook for a further 1½ minutes. Stir in the prawns and leave for 1½ minutes. Refresh noodles with boiling water, pour into a serving dish and spoon the chow mein on top.

Baked gammon pot   ◆ W M E

Serves 4–6

1.5 kg/3 lb approx gammon joint
1 stick celery, chopped
1 large carrot, chopped
1 leek, sliced
1 tbsp parsley
1 bay-leaf
2 or 3 whole cloves garlic
1 tsp demerara sugar

Put the gammon in a bowl, cover with cold water and leave to soak for 2–4 hours or overnight. Rinse in fresh cold water, place in a saucepan, cover with cold water and bring to the boil. Allow to boil for 2 minutes, drain, rinse with cold water and put in a casserole.

Add the vegetables, parsley, bay-leaf, garlic and sugar. Cover with water, place in the oven and bake at 160°C/325°F/Gas Mark 3 for 20 minutes per 450 g/lb plus 20 minutes, or until cooked.

Remove from the oven, keep covered and leave to rest in a warm place for 20 minutes. Serve hot or cold.

Somerset pork casserole   ◆ⓦⓜⒺ

Serves 4

4 pork fillets or 565 g/1¼ lb pork pieces
1 tbsp sunflower oil
1 medium leek, chopped
2 sticks celery, chopped
170 ml/6 fl oz apple juice or white grape juice
2–3 tbsp water
generous pinch dried sage or, preferably, 1 tsp fresh sage,
    chopped
1 clove garlic, crushed
salt and pepper
30 g/1 oz arrowroot
2 tbsp soya cream

Heat the oil in a pan, add the fillets or pieces of pork and
sauté until sealed and beginning to brown. Remove to a casserole. Cook the leek and celery in the pan in the same oil for
4–5 minutes until beginning to soften, but do not allow to
brown. Remove and add to the casserole.

Pour the water and apple or grape juice into the pan. Add
the sage and garlic, season to taste and bring to the boil.
Remove from the heat.

Mix the arrowroot with a little water. Add 2 tbsp of hot
stock from the pan and mix well, then pour back into the pan.
Return to the heat and simmer for 2 minutes, until the liquid
has thickened.

Pour into the casserole and bake at 180°C/350°F°C/Gas
Mark 4 for 40–45 minutes. Remove from the oven, stir in the
cream and serve.

Chilli pork ragout ◆WME

Serves 4

450 g/1 lb pork pieces
2 tbsp sunflower oil
225–280 g/8–10 oz (dry weight) long-grain rice, cooked
140 g/5 oz celery, finely chopped
170 g/6 oz red kidney beans, cooked
1 small green pepper, cut into chunks
1 small red pepper, cut into chunks
3 spikes chives, chopped
1/2 tsp dried basil
1/2 tsp ground ginger
1/2 tsp turmeric
1/2 tsp chilli powder, or to taste
170 ml/6 fl oz good stock (see page 143)
salt and pepper

In a large pan or wok, heat the oil and sauté the pork pieces until lightly golden and just tender. Remove from the pan and keep warm.

In the same pan, cook the celery, beans, peppers, chives, spices and stock over a gentle heat until the vegetables are just tender. Return the pork to the pan and cook until it is heated through and the moisture is absorbed.

Pour boiling water through the rice to warm and serve with the chilli ragout.

Orchard pork chops ◆WME

Serves 2

2 pork chops, trimmed and seasoned
1/2 large cooking apple or 1 medium apple, peeled, cored
    and chopped
1 pear, peeled, cored and chopped
2 whole cloves garlic
1 small tsp demerara sugar
salt

Line an ovenproof dish with tin foil, leaving enough on the sides to fold over. Lay the chops in the dish.

Put the apple and pear in a saucepan adding the sugar and a little water. Cook over a medium heat until the fruit is pulped. Remove the from heat and strain.

Add the juice to the chops, sprinkle with cloves and add a little water and a pinch of salt. Fold the foil over the chops and bake at 180°C/350°F/Gas Mark 4 for 30–40 minutes.

Pork and pineapple grill

Serves 4

4 lean pork chops
1 tbsp sunflower oil
340 g/12 oz spinach, fresh or frozen
salt and pepper
4 pineapple rings (one small tin)
1 dessertspoon pine nuts, toasted
1 dessertspoon sunflower seeds, toasted
pinch nutmeg

Heat the grill pan, brush both sides of the chops with oil, season and place under the grill. Grill for 8–10 minutes, depending on the thickness of the meat, brushing often with oil. Turn the chops and cook for a further 8 minutes. Remove from the pan and keep warm.

Drain the pineapple, brush with oil and grill both sides until lightly golden. Put the spinach in a hot pan with 2 tsp of oil and a pinch of nutmeg. Sweat, stirring continuously, for 2–3 minutes, until the spinach is wilting,

Remove from the pan and put in the base of warm dish. Lay the pork chops on top, place a pineapple ring on each chop and sprinkle toasted nuts and seeds over the whole dish.

CHRISTMAS

Almost a punch

Serves 3

600 ml/1 pt pure red grape juice
little demerara sugar to taste
2 cloves and 2 good pinches cinnamon
260 ml/^{1}/$_{2}$ pint juice

Put all the ingredients in a pan, gently warm through to medium heat, strain and serve in warmed glasses.

Festive salmon mousse

Serves 4

150 ml (^{1}/4 pt) aspic jelly
few mint leaves
few slices cucumber
30 g/1 oz dairy-free margarine
30 g/1 oz gram flour (or any suitable flour used for thickening)
300 ml/^{1}/$_{2}$ pint soya milk
220 g/7^{3}/4 oz tin pink salmon
100 g/3^{1}/2 oz soya cream
salt and pepper
15 g/^{1}/2 oz vegetable gelatine

Make up the aspic jelly as directed. Rinse a round 15 cm/6 in cake tin with cold water, pour half the aspic jelly into the base and leave it in a cool place to set.

Wash and dry the mint leaves. Dip the mint leaves and cucumber in the aspic jelly and arrange them decoratively on the set jelly in the tin. Leave to set. Then pour on the remaining aspic and leave to set.

Melt the margarine in a pan, stir in the flour for 2 minutes, then remove from the heat Stir in the milk, return to the heat and bring to the boil, stirring constantly. Simmer for 2 minutes.

Drain the salmon and remove any skin and bones. Stir the salmon and cream into the sauce and season to taste.

Dissolve the gelatine in 2 tbsp cold water and stir into the salmon mixture. Allow to cool. Pour salmon mixture into tin and allow to set in refrigerator.

When ready to serve, dip the tin in hot water for a few seconds, turn onto a plate and garnish.

Stuffed turkey breast

Serves 6–8

breast of turkey, 1½–2½kg/3½–5 lb in weight
280 g/10 oz unsmoked lean bacon
2 leeks, washed and cut into fine rings
2–3 level tsp oregano
sunflower oil

Open out the breast of turkey, wipe clean and trim off any odd pieces of skin. Beat any extra-thick parts with a rolling pin until the meat is a fairly even thickness all over.

Trim the bacon and lay rashers across the turkey to line the inside. Scatter rings of leeks all over and sprinkle the oregano over the leeks. Roll up the breast lengthways and tie at intervals with string.

Place the turkey on a sheet of baking foil and brush well with oil. Fold the foil over to loosely enclose it. Bake for approximately 20 mins/lb plus an extra 20 minutes at 190°C/375°F/Gas Mark 5, reducing to 180°C/340°F/Gas Mark 4 after the first hour, brushing at intervals. Open up the foil for the last 30 minutes and allow the turkey to brown.

Pork fillet with spiced peaches and cream

Serves 4

450 g/1 lb pork fillet, trimmed and prepared
salt and freshly ground black pepper
2 or 3 large peaches (450 g/1 lb in weight approx)
225–280 ml/8–10 fl oz white grape juice
60 g/2 oz caster sugar
2 whole cloves garlic
2 whole allspice
25 mm/1 in piece cinnamon stick
1 tsp rice vinegar
little soya cream

Season the pork fillet and loosely wrap it in lightly greased oven foil. Place in a roasting tin and cook for 30–40 minutes or until the juices run clear and meat is tender, at 180°C/350°F/Gas Mark 4.

Meanwhile, plunge the peaches into boiling water and skin them. Slice each peach in half and then each half into three. Put the grape juice, sugar, garlic, spices and vinegar in a saucepan and bring to the boil. Simmer for 10 minutes, then spoon the peach slices into the syrup and simmer for a further 5–6 minutes. Remove the peaches and keep warm. Boil the syrup to reduce by about a third to a half.

Remove from the heat, discard the garlic and spices and add the juices from the pork to the remaining syrup. Swirl in some soya cream. Spoon a little of the spiced cream syrup onto each plate and add slices of pork fillet with peach slices arranged between.

The Christmas ham

Serves 4–6

1–1½kg/2–3 lb joint of gammon
2 tbsp clear honey
1 large mango, stone removed and flesh chopped
little pineapple juice
pinch of either allspice or cinnamon or cloves (optional)

The day before cooking, rinse the gammon in cold water, put in a large bowl, cover with cold water and leave overnight.

Next day, remove from the bowl and rinse with fresh clean water. Put the joint in a saucepan, cover with cold water, bring to the boil and boil for 2 minutes. Drain and rinse with cold water again; this should remove all excess salt.

Dry the gammon and place it on a large sheet of foil. Spread a thin covering of honey over the surface of the gammon and bake at 160°C//325°F/Gas Mark 3 for half the required cooking time (total cooking time approx 20 mins/lb plus an extra 20 minutes), basting in the juices at intervals. Remove from the oven, open the foil and add the chopped mango to the gammon. Pour over the pineapple juice, sprinkle over the pinch of spice if using, re-wrap the joint and return it to oven, basting frequently.

Thirty minutes before the end of the cooking time, open the foil and allow the gammon to become lightly golden. Do not let the mango over-brown.

Celery and tomato stuffing

Serves 2–3

170 g/6 oz cooked white rice
60 g/2 oz celery, chopped finely
2 tomatoes, skinned, seeded and chopped
2 tsp mixed herbs
salt and pepper to taste
1 egg white, beaten, or 1–2 tbsp dairy-free margarine, melted

Combine all the ingredients except the last, adding the egg white or melted margarine to bring the mixture together.

Leek, mushroom and apple stuffing   ◆W◆ ◆M◆

Serves 2

115 g/4 oz cooked brown rice
60 g/2 oz leeks, cut into fine rings
60 g/2 oz chestnut or button mushrooms, chopped
60 g/2 oz stewed apple
salt and pepper
1 egg white, beaten

Combine the first four ingredients in a bowl, season to taste, add the egg white and mix well. If the mixture is too stiff, add a spoonful of hot water.

A pudding to enjoy   ◆W◆ ◆M◆

Serves 6–8

115 g/4 oz flour mix (see page 158)
115 g/4 oz wheat-free soda breadcrumbs (see page 160)
225 g/8 oz soft dark brown sugar
pinch salt
pinch nutmeg
225 ml/8 fl oz sunflower oil (preferably 'buttery' variety)
225 g/8 oz currants
225 g/8 oz raisins
225 g/8 oz sultanas
2 large eggs
150 ml/¼ pint soya milk
60 g/2 oz toasted pine nuts
little rum or brandy to taste (optional)

Mix all the ingredients together except the rum or brandy (if using), then stir in the liquor and leave to stand overnight.

Mix again and spoon into a 1.5l/3½ pt basin. Cover with double thickness of grease-proof paper and then tin foil. Steam for at least 6–8 hours.

The longer you steam this pudding, the tastier it will be.

Christmas cake

For a 18–20 cm/7–8 in cake tin

225 g/8 oz high-fibre flour mix, mixed with 60 g/2 oz
 wheat-free baking powder (see page 158)
1/2 tsp natural pectin or 2 tsp xanthan gum
1 tsp mixed spice
pinch cinnamon
115 g/4 oz soft dark brown sugar
1 tbsp black treacle
340 g/12 oz mixed currants, sultanas, raisins
60 g/2 oz glacé cherries, washed and chopped
few drops almond essence
2 large eggs, beaten
115 ml/4 fl oz sunflower oil (preferably 'buttery' variety)
115 ml/4 fl oz soya milk

Sift the flour and baking powder into a bowl, then stir in the
powdered pectin, spices, sugar, dried fruit and cherries.

 Mix together the beaten eggs, treacle, oil, milk and almond
essence. Add to the dry ingredients and mix to an even dropping consistency.

 Bake in greased and lined 18–20 cm/7–8 in cake tin at
150°C/325°F/Gas Mark 3 for 1 1/2–1 3/4 hours, or until cooked.

Eggless festive cake

For a 20 cm/8 in cake tin

225 g/8 oz flour mix and 2 tsp wheat-free baking powder
 (see page 158), sifted together
1 tsp mixed spice
pinch nutmeg
170 g/6 oz mixed currants, sultanas, raisins
60 g/2 oz glacé cherries, washed and chopped
200 ml/7 fl oz soya milk
340 g/12 oz golden syrup
225 g/8 oz dairy-free margarine, melted
few drops vanilla essence
1/2 tsp natural pectin or 2 tsp xanthan gum

Stir the golden syrup into melted margarine and add the vanilla essence. Mix together all the dry ingredients, and then add the milk, margarine and syrup mixture.

Spoon into greased and lined 20 cm/8 in cake tin and bake at 130°C/300°F/Gas Mark 2 for 1–1½ hours, or until cooked.

When cool, double wrap the cake (one layer of greaseproof and one layer of foil), place it in an airtight container and leave for at least a week.

Mincemeat of a kind

115 g/4 oz sultanas
115 g/4 oz raisins
85 g/3 oz glacé cherries, washed free of sugar
60 g/2 oz dried, ready-to-eat apricots
85 g/3 oz eating apple, grated
2 tbsp white grape juice
1 tsp clear honey
1 tsp cinnamon
1 tsp allspice
pinch nutmeg
2 tbsp brandy or rum (optional, but it does help to preserve)
1 tbsp toasted pine nuts

Mince or finely chop the fruits and put into a bowl. Put the grape juice, honey, spices and brandy/rum (if using) into a small pan. Bring to the boil and simmer for 2 minutes. Remove from the heat.

Pour into a clean jug to cool quickly. When just warm, pour over the fruits and mix thoroughly, but do not beat. Adjust the quantity of liquid at this stage. Finally, fold in the pine nuts.

Spoon into clean, sterile jars, with tight-fitting lids. Stored in the refrigerator, this mincemeat will keep for 3–4 weeks.

Mincemeat pie filling

170 g/6 oz chopped apples and pears
255 g/9 oz mixed dried fruit
30 g/1 oz glacé cherries, chopped
few drops vanilla essence
85 g/3 oz soft brown sugar (molasses is good)
1 tsp cinnamon
good pinch of nutmeg
2 tbsp white grape or pineapple juice
85 ml/3 fl oz brandy (omit for exclusion diet)

Put all the ingredients in a pan and simmer over a low heat for 35–40 minutes, stirring frequently. Allow to cool, pack into clean, sterile jars, seal and store in the refrigerator.

STOCKS AND SAUCES

Stock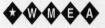

If you make your own stock you can be sure that it is appropriate for your allowed diet. It is also inexpensive, and is to hand whenever you need it.

The basic ingredients for a good stock are:

1 large carrot
1 leek
1 or 2 sticks celery
bouquet garni

To this add fish bones, chicken carcass or beef bones. Cover with water, add salt and pepper and bring to the boil. Skim off any scum that may appear, reduce to the lowest heat and allow the pot to simmer slowly for 2–3 hours. Do not be tempted to stir the contents of the pan – this would give you a cloudy stock.

Turn off the heat, remove the pan from the cooker and leave the stock to rest until just warm. Strain to remove vegetables, bones and bouquet garni. Allow to become cold and skim off any fat that may have settled. Pour into suitable containers and freeze.

Vegetable stock

The most economical way of making vegetable stock is to save usable vegetable trimmings when preparing vegetables for meals. Put them into a covered tub in the refrigerator. They will keep for a couple of days.

Rinse the vegetables/trimmings, put them in a pan with a handful of fresh mixed herbs and cover with salted water. Bring to the boil and simmer for 1–1½ hours. Strain the liquid from the vegetables and leave to cool. Spoon into suitable containers and freeze.

For convenience, you can use some of the commercial alternatives that are available. Supermarkets produce their own fresh stocks, although chicken stock tends to be the only one suitable for the exclusion diet (check ingredients carefully). Some stock cubes and powders are available from health-food shops that are wheat-, dairy- and yeast-free.

Curry salad dressing

225 ml/8 fl oz soya yoghurt
2 tsp korma curry powder (check ingredients carefully)
2 level tsp tomato purée
60 ml/2 fl oz pineapple juice

Mix all the ingredients together thoroughly until blended. Keep refrigerated.

Mushroom sauce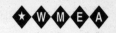

225 g/8 oz mushrooms, wiped and chopped
30 g/1 oz sunflower oil or dairy-free margarine
280–340 g/10–12 oz beef or chicken stock (see page 143)
1 heaped tsp fresh mixed herbs, finely chopped
little arrowroot if necessary
salt and pepper

Heat the oil in a pan or wok, add the mushrooms and cook for 2–3 minutes. Add the stock and herbs, bring to the boil and lower the heat to a simmer for 5–6 minutes.

Set aside 1 tsp of chopped mushrooms, transfer remaining contents to liquidizer and blend.

Return to the pan and add the reserved mushrooms. Reheat, thickening with a little arrowroot if necessary.

Savoury white sauce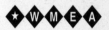

300 ml/½ pint soya milk
15 g/½ oz dairy-free margarine
salt
4–6 black peppercorns
2 tsp wheat-free Dijon mustard (or 2 tbsp fresh chives or
    parsley, chopped)
little arrowroot to thicken
small bay-leaf

Put the milk, margarine, salt to taste, black peppercorns, and bay-leaf in a saucepan. Heat over a very low heat until hot, but not boiling.

Remove from the heat and leave to infuse for 30 minutes. Remove the bay-leaf and peppercorns and stir in the Dijon mustard or herbs. Mix the arrowroot with a little cold soya milk, add 2 tbsp warm soya milk and return to the saucepan.

Mix well and return to the heat. Bring to the boil, stirring, then simmer for 2 minutes.

Herb dressing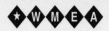

170–280 ml/6–10 fl oz light olive oil, depending on amount
    you wish to make
2–3 tbsp apple juice or white grape juice
2 tbsp fresh chives, chopped
2 tbsp fresh parsley, chopped
1 tbsp fresh dill, chopped
salt to taste

Add the herbs to the juice and whisk well together. Gradually
add the oil, drop by drop, whisking continuously. Transfer to
a screw-top container and refrigerate until required.

Mint and cucumber
yogurt sauce

300 ml/¹/₂ pint soya yoghurt
2 tsp fresh chives, finely chopped
1 tbsp fresh mint leaves, chopped
1 heaped tbsp cucumber, chopped
salt to taste

Whisk all the ingredients together in a bowl and refrigerate
until needed.
    This sauce is ideal for curries.

Hasty tomato and mushroom
sauce

1 stick celery, chopped
1–2 tbsp olive oil
115 g/4 oz mushrooms, sliced
400 g/14 oz jar of sieved or tinned tomatoes, drained

2 tbsp tomato purée
2 tsp chives, chopped
pinch each oregano, thyme and basil
1 small bay-leaf
salt and pepper

Cook the celery in the oil for 2–3 minutes, then add the mushrooms, tomatoes, purée, herbs and seasoning. Simmer on a very low heat for 10 minutes. Remove the bay-leaf, and serve as required.

Lentil apple sauce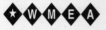

115 g/4 oz lentils, washed, soaked and ready to cook
850 ml/1¹/₂ pints vegetable stock (see page 144)
garni of chives, thyme and a small bay-leaf
1–2 tbsp sunflower oil
2 large carrots, chopped
1 large stick celery, finely sliced
1 large Cox's apple (a Bramley can be used), peeled, cored
   and chopped
salt and pepper

Cook the lentils in the stock for 30–40 minutes with the herb garni. Heat the oil in a frying pan, add the carrots and celery and cook for about 5 minutes over a low heat. Then add the apple.

Continue cooking until the carrots and celery are cooked. Transfer to a blender, add the lentils and blend well. Season to taste with salt and pepper.

Alternatively, run the sauce through a sieve until smooth.

DESSERTS

Gingered pears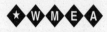

Serves 6

6 firm pears
225 ml/8 fl oz white grape juice
25 mm/1 in piece of fresh ginger, peeled and cut into three
   pieces
little soya cream
chopped stem ginger to garnish

Peel the pears, leaving the stems on, and slice across the
bottoms so that the pears stand up.

Place the pears in a saucepan, pour over the grape juice and
add the ginger. Cover and cook over a low heat until the pears
are just tender. Remove from the heat and leave to cool.

To serve, remove the ginger and place the pears in individual dishes, spooning a little juice over them. Pour a little soya
cream around the base of each pear and sprinkle a little
chopped stem ginger into the cream.

Apple and sultana brulée

Serves 2

3 medium apples, peeled, cored and chopped
85 g/3 oz sultanas
brown sugar to taste
2 tbsp water
2 x 120 g/4 oz cartons soya yoghurt
brown sugar

Put the apples, sugar and water in a pan and poach until the
apples are tender. Stir in the sultanas and poach for a further
5 minutes, until the liquid has reduced.

Divide the fruit between two individual dishes and empty a

carton of yoghurt into each dish. Sprinkle a layer of brown sugar over the top and place under a hot grill until the sugar caramelizes.

The brulée can be served on its own or with a piece of shortbread (see page 164)

Pear and raspberry crumble

Serves 4

2 medium pears, peeled, cored and sliced
115 g/4 oz raspberries, washed
little sugar if necessary

Crumble topping:
115 g/4 oz high-fibre flour mix (see page 158)
60 g/2 oz dairy-free margarine
40 g/1½ oz caster sugar
1 tsp cinnamon

Poach the fruit until it begins to soften, adding sugar if required, then place in a basin or ovenproof dish.

Rub the fat into the flour to a breadcrumb consistency. Stir in the sugar and cinnamon until evenly mixed and spoon over the fruit.

Bake for 20–25 minutes, or until golden brown, at 180°C/350°F/Gas Mark 4.

Banana and sultana pudding

Serves 2

600 ml/1 pint soya milk
60 g/2 oz caster sugar
60 g/2 oz flaked rice
60 g/2 oz sultanas
pinch cinnamon
2 bananas
2 heaped tbsp demerara sugar

Put the milk, sugar, rice, sultanas and cinnamon in a saucepan. Bring slowly to the boil, stirring frequently. Lower the heat and simmer for 12–15 minutes, until thick.

Pour into a suitable heat-proof dish. Slice the bananas thinly and lay over the top. Cover with a thick layer of sugar. Brown under the grill.

Serve hot or cold with a little soya cream if wished.

Moreish pear and apricot quickie

Serves 4

280 g/10 oz pears, peeled, cored and sliced
225 g/8 oz dried, ready-to-eat apricots, halved
225 ml/8 fl oz water
1 large tbsp honey
pinch cinnamon
pinch ground cloves (optional)
1 1/2 heaped tbsp brown sugar
1 tbsp pine nuts

Put the pears, apricots, water, honey and spices in a saucepan over a gentle heat and poach until the fruit is tender.

Remove the fruit to a suitable ovenproof dish, increase the heat and boil the poaching liquid until thick and syrupy. Pour over the fruit, spoon the sugar over the top and sprinkle with pine nuts. Place under a hot grill until the sugar has caramelized and the pine nuts are toasted.

Pear condé

Serves 4

600 ml/1 pint soya milk
30 g/1 oz caster sugar
85 g/3 oz pudding rice, washed
few drops vanilla essence

8 pear halves, poached until tender, or canned in natural
   juices
4 tbsp apricot jam
120 ml/4 oz carton soya yoghurt

Put the milk, sugar, rice and vanilla essence in an ovenproof
dish and bake in a slow oven for 1¹/₂–2 hours, stirring
occasionally.

When the rice is cooked and most of the milk has been
absorbed, remove, leave until cool, then chill in the refrigerator.

Divide the rice pudding between four bowls and lay the
pear halves on top, cut side down. Warm the apricot jam and
use it to brush the pears and rice well.

Spoon over a thickish topping of soya yoghurt, make a
swirl in the yoghurt with a fork and serve.

Simply super sweet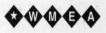

Serves 1

mixture of fresh mango, pineapple and paw-paw (papaya),
   sliced (to individual taste)
sunflower oil (preferably 'buttery' variety)
ground ginger to taste
few drops vanilla essence

Heat the grill to medium-high, line the grill pan with tin foil
and lay the fruit in layers on the foil.

Pour a little sunflower oil into a small bowl. Add 2–3 drops
of vanilla essence. Brush well over fruit and sprinkle with
ground ginger.

Place under the grill until bubbling and lightly golden.
Then turn the fruit over and repeat on the other side.

Serve with soya yoghurt or, for a special treat, liquidize a
slice of ripe melon and add 1 tsp medium-sweet white wine to
serve with it as a sauce.

Taste of Jamaica

Serves 4

wheat-free pastry using 225 g/8 oz flour mix (see page 165)
2 bananas, sliced
1/2 large mango, chopped
115 g/4 oz golden syrup
60 g/2 oz wheat-free breadcrumbs or wheat-free sponge cake
    crumbs (see pages 160 & 173)
1/2 tsp ground ginger

Line a greased 18–20 cm/7–8 inch pie plate with the pastry, reserving enough to make a top. Cover the base with a mixture of mango and banana.

Stir the crumbs and ground ginger into the golden syrup and spoon over the fruit. Roll out the remaining pastry and cover the pie.

Bake at 180°C/350°F/Gas Mark 4 for 25–30 minutes, or until the pastry is cooked and the top is golden brown. This dessert may take a little effort, but it is certainly worth it!

Pancake mixture

Serves 4

115 g/4 oz flour mix (see page 158)
pinch salt
1 egg
85 ml/3 fl oz soya milk plus 85 ml/3 fl oz water
1 tbsp sunflower oil

Sift the flour and salt together in a bowl. Make a well in the centre, put in the egg and a little of the milk and beat really well until smoothly blended. Gradually add the remaining liquid until you have a smooth batter of a creamy consistency. Leave in a cool place for 20 minutes. Add 1 tbsp oil and beat for 2 minutes, then leave to rest for 10 minutes.

Heat the remaining oil in a frying pan. When very hot, whisk the batter and pour in the required amount. Cook over a fairly high heat. When the edges are curling and golden, turn the pancake and cook the remaining batter in the same way.

The pancakes can be used for either sweet or savoury fillings.

Summer pudding

Serves 6

sponge mixture made with 170 g/6 oz flour mix and wheat-
   free baking powder (see pages 159 & 173)
1 large cooking apple, peeled, cored, and chopped
450 g/1 lb red fruit, e.g. plums, berries
sugar to taste
115 g/4 fl oz water

Grease and line a swiss-roll tin, pour in the sponge mixture and bake. Remove from the oven and cool.

Meanwhile, put the apple in a saucepan with some sugar and the water and cook for 15–20 minutes. Add the other fruit and continue cooking until all the fruit is soft. Remove from the heat and set aside to cool.

Cut two-thirds of the sponge into wedges and line a glass or ceramic basin. Pour in the fruit mixture and cut the remainder of the sponge to fit the top as a lid. Place a saucer or plate on top and weigh it down. Leave in the refrigerator overnight.

Serve with soya cream or soya yoghurt.

Bread pudding

Serves 6

Wheat-free bread loaf using 450 g/1 lb flour mix (see page 160)

300 ml/^{1}/$_2$ pint soya milk

1 large egg, beaten

115 g/4 oz sugar, preferably moist brown sugar

225 g/8 oz dried fruit, mixed

1 tsp mixed spice

^{1}/$_4$ tsp cinnamon

Cut the bread into cubes and soak in the milk until the liquid has been absorbed. Stir to make sure there are no lumps.

Add all the remaining ingredients, mixing well to combine. The mixture should not be too wet.

Spoon into a greased and lined 5 cm/2 in deep rectangular cake tin (18–20 cm/7–8 inch square). Sprinkle a mixture of brown sugar and cinnamon over the top and bake in at 180°C/350°F/Gas Mark 4 for 1–1^1/$_4$ hours, or until cooked and firm to the touch.

Baked banana sponge

Serves 4

115 g/4 oz high-fibre flour mix plus 1 tsp wheat-free baking powder sifted together (see page 158)

85 g/3 oz dairy-free margarine

60 g/2 oz caster sugar

vanilla essence

2 small eggs, beaten

2 small bananas, sliced

Cream the margarine and sugar until pale and fluffy. Add a few drops of vanilla essence to the beaten eggs and stir a little into the creamed mixture along with 1 tbsp of the flour mix.

Gradually add the remaining egg, sliced bananas and 1 tbsp of flour mix to combine. Fold in the remaining flour mix.

Transfer to greased and lined 450 g/1 lb loaf tin and bake for 20 minutes at 180°C/350°F/Gas Mark 4. Reduce the oven temperature to 160°C/325°F/Gas Mark 3 and bake for a further 20 minutes, or until the sponge is cooked.

Serve with soya custard or soya yoghurt.

Apple cake pudding

Serves 6

225 g/8 oz flour mix plus 2 tsp wheat-free baking powder, sifted together (see page 158)
115 g/4 oz dairy-free margarine
115 g/4 oz caster sugar
1 egg, beaten
1 medium–large apple, peeled, cored and grated
1/2 tsp vanilla essence
soya milk
little demerara sugar

Beat the margarine and sugar together until pale and fluffy. Add the beaten egg, vanilla essence and a little flour. Gradually beat in the rest of the flour and add the grated apple. Add sufficient milk to reach a dropping consistency.

Bake at 180°C/350°F/Gas Mark 4 for about 1 hour, or until cooked. This makes an excellent pudding served with soya custard.

Pineapple upside-down pudding

Serves 6

340 g/12 oz pineapple rings, drained
6 glacé cherries
170 g/6 oz flour mix and 11/2 tsp wheat-free baking powder sifted together (see page 158)
115 g/4 oz dairy-free margarine
60 g/2 oz caster sugar
2 large eggs, beaten
1 tbsp soya milk

Wash the cherries free of their sugar coating, dry and cut into halves. Dry the pineapple rings using kitchen paper.

Lightly grease and line an 18 cm/7 in cake tin. Put a pineapple ring in the centre of the tin and arrange the remaining rings around it. Place a cherry in the centre of each pineapple ring.

Cream the margarine and sugar until pale and fluffy. Add the egg a little at a time, adding a spoonful of flour with the first quantity of egg. Fold in the remaining flour/baking powder mix. Add the milk to give a dropping consistency.

Spoon the mixture over the pineapple rings, covering them completely. Bake for 40–45 minutes at 180°C/350°F/Gas Mark 4. Remove from the oven and leave to stand for a few minutes before turning out onto a dish. Serve hot or cold.

Blackcurrant and tofu whip   ★ W M E

Serves 4–6

450 g/1 lb ripe blackcurrants
sugar to taste
280 g/10 oz tofu

Put the blackcurrants in a pan with a little water and sugar to taste. Bring to the boil and stew until the blackcurrants are tender. Leave to cool. Place in a blender with the tofu and liquidize until smooth. Chill well before serving.

Note: other fruits such as blackberries or gooseberries can be substituted for the blackcurrants in this recipe.

Carob ice-cream

Serves 4–6

60 g/2 oz runny honey
500 ml/18 fl oz soya milk
4 tbsp sunflower oil
1/4 tsp salt
60 g/2 oz carob powder

Put all the ingredients in a blender and liquidize until smooth. Pour into a suitable container and freeze for approximately 3 hours, until the mixture begins to set. Beat with a fork, then return to the freezer to firm up for at least 1 hour.

Transfer to the refrigerator 30 minutes before serving, to allow the ice-cream to soften.

Note: This ice-cream can be made with other flavourings besides carob powder, such as puréed fruit.

Apricot mould

Serves 4

130 g/41/2 oz dried apricots
2 tbsp granulated sugar
1 sachet powdered gelatine (about 15 g/1/2 oz)

Pour boiling water over 100 g/31/2 oz of the apricots and leave to soak for several hours. Drain and wash. Stew for 10 minutes, until soft, in 60 ml/2 fl oz water. Sieve to make a purée, then stir in the sugar.

Dissolve the gelatine in 90 ml/3 fl oz very hot water, stirring briskly. Make up to 300 ml/1/2 pint with cold water, then stir into the apricot mixture.

Arrange the remaining dried apricots on the base of a wetted mould, then carefully pour in the mixture. Allow to set in a refrigerator for 3 hours.

BAKING

Flour mixes

The gluten-free flour mixes you can buy are usually unsuitable for exclusion diets because they contain wheat starch, corn (or maize) flour, potato flour or a combination of these. They also tend to be expensive as they are prescribable only for those with confirmed Coeliac disease.

Substituting a single alternative flour, e.g. rice flour, for normal wheat flour gives disappointing results when baking because gluten is essential for the light, doughy consistency we associate with bread. However, this characteristic can be mimicked using a combination of flours and a binding agent such as guar gum, xanthan gum or pectin. These flours and binders should all be available from a good health-food shop.

The following mixes are all suitable for wheat-, milk- and egg-free diets. The recipes containing amaranth flour are also suitable for exclusion and arthritis exclusion diets. Amaranth flour gives particularly good results. It has a nutty flavour and when mixed with a high-starch grain flour gives a good texture and retains moisture. Unfortunately, it is not as readily available as other flours.

For bread, lighter cakes, pastry and scones choose from recipes A to D. A high-fibre flour mix can be made by adding rice bran to these (recipe E). Recipe F is more suitable for heavier cakes such as fruit cakes and some savoury dishes.

A   225 g/8 oz amaranth flour   ★ⓌⓂⒺⒶ
     450 g/1 lb rice flour
     30 g/1 oz binder (guar gum, xanthan gum or pectin)

B   675 g/1½ lb amaranth flour   ★ⓌⓂⒺⒶ
     225 g/8 oz tapioca flour
     30 g/1 oz binder (as above)

C   85 g/3 oz tapioca flour
     60 g/2 oz soya flour
     60 g/2 oz rice flour
     30 g/1 oz cornflour
     15 g/¹/₂ oz binder (as above)

D   85 g/3 oz rice flour
     85 g/3 oz tapioca flour
     60 g/2 oz farina (potato starch)
     15 g/¹/₂ oz binder (as above)

E   For **high-fibre** flour, add 1 tbsp finely ground rice bran
     to any of the above mixes.

A to E: suitable for bread, lighter cakes, pastry, scones, etc.
Blend all the ingredients together well. Store in an airtight
plastic container.

F   510 g/1 lb 2 oz fine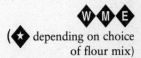
        ground rice flour
     85 g/4 oz soya flour
     60 g/2 oz gram flour
     225 g/8 oz polenta or desiccated coconut (this must be
        very finely ground in processor) or 225 g/8 oz ground
        almonds
     30 g/1 oz binder (guar gum, xanthan gum or pectin)

Suitable for heavier cakes such as fruit cakes and some savoury
dishes. Blend all the ingredients together well. Store in an
airtight plastic container. Makes approximately 900 g/2 lb.

Wheat-free baking powder

As these flour mixes are very light compared to wheat flour, baking powder works better as a raising agent than yeast. Commercial wheat-free brands are available from health-food shops and
some supermarkets, but a cheaper version can be home-made.

170 g/6 oz tapioca or rice flour
200 g/7 oz bicarbonate of soda or potassium bicarbonate
85 g/4 oz cream of tartar
60 g/2 oz tartaric acid

Sieve all the ingredients together and store in an airtight container. Sieve the required amount again just before use.

Soda bread

450 g/16 oz high-fibre flour mix (see page 158)
260 ml/1/2 pint soya milk
2 egg whites, beaten
1/4 tsp salt
1 heaped tsp bicarbonate of soda or potassium bicarbonate
1 heaped tsp cream of tartar
30 g/1 oz sesame seeds

Place the flour, salt, bicarbonate of soda and cream of tartar in a bowl. Add the liquid ingredients, stirring well, until a smooth, thick batter is achieved.

Place the batter in a well-greased 900 g/2 lb loaf tin. Brush the top with oil and sprinkle the sesame seeds on top.

Bake at 180°C/350°F/Gas Mark 4 for 40–45 minutes or until well risen and firm to the touch.

Tomato and basil soda bread

450 g/16 oz high-fibre flour mix (see page 158)
260 ml/1/2 pint water
2 egg whites, beaten
1/4 tsp salt
1 heaped tsp bicarbonate of soda or potassium bicarbonate
1 heaped tsp cream of tartar
60 g/2 oz dried tomatoes

3–4 drops pure basil oil
2 level tbsp fresh basil leaves, torn into pieces
poppy seeds to sprinkle

Soak the dried tomatoes in boiling water for 20 minutes.
Drain and dry well and cut into small strips.

Place the flour, salt, bicarbonate of soda and cream of
tartar in a bowl. Add the tomato slices and torn basil leaves
and stir. Stir the basil oil into the egg and add with water to
the dry ingredients. Beat to a smooth but thick batter.

Place the batter in a greased 20 cm/8 in sandwich tin lined
with baking paper. Mark a cross in the batter. Brush with oil
and sprinkle with poppy seeds.

Bake at 180°C/350°F/Gas Mark 4 for 40–45 minutes or
until well risen and firm to the touch.

Chapattis

Makes 10 approx   (✦ depending on choice of flour mix)
200 g/7 oz high-fibre flour mix (see page 158)
30 g/1 oz rice bran
1/4 tsp salt
30 g/1 oz dairy-free margarine
150 ml/1/4 pint water
sunflower oil for frying

Mix the flour, bran and salt in a bowl. Add the margarine and
rub into a breadcrumb consistency. Add water to mix to a stiff
dough.

Knead well on a floured board for 5 minutes. Leave to rest
for 20 minutes. Divide the dough into ten pieces and roll out
each piece into a circle.

Heat the oil in a frying pan and fry each chapatti for 3
minutes, turning frequently. Serve warm.

Sweet potato bread

Makes 16 pieces   (◆ depending on choice of flour mix)

225 g/8 oz sweet potato, scrubbed but not peeled
170 g/6 oz flour mix (see page 158)
pinch salt
pinch nutmeg
pinch cumin
sunflower oil for frying

Cook the potatoes in boiling water for 8–10 minutes. Drain and rinse them in cold water, then remove peel and grate into a bowl.

Add the flour, salt and spices to the potato and mix to a soft dough. Add a little cold water if necessary. Divide the dough into sixteen pieces and dust with flour. Roll each piece on a floured board.

Heat the oil in heavy frying pan and shallow fry the bread pieces, a few at a time, for 2–3 minutes. Drain on kitchen paper.

Baker's scones

Makes 6–8 scones   (◆ depending on choice of flour mix)

115 g/4 oz high-fibre flour mix (see page 158)
115 g/4 oz flour mix
or
200 g/7 oz flour mix and
30 g/1 oz pure rice bran

2 tsp wheat-free baking powder (see page 159)
30 g/1 oz caster sugar
60 g/2 oz dairy-free margarine
140 g/5 oz soya milk
1/2 tsp vanilla essence
pinch salt

Place the flour in a clean bowl, add the salt and baking powder and mix well. Add the margarine and rub in until it resembles fine breadcrumbs. Stir in the sugar.

Add the vanilla essence to the milk and stir. Add to the dry ingredients and mix to a soft but not sticky consistency. Add a little more milk if necessary, but avoid making the mixture too wet.

Flour a board and gently roll the mixture to a good 25 mm/1 in thickness. Cut out the scones and place on a greased baking sheet. Brush the tops with egg or milk if desired.

Bake in the oven for about 10 minutes at 220°C/425°F/Gas Mark 7 or until lightly golden. Leave them to cool, then place them on a wire rack until cold.

Derby scones

Makes 6–8 scones   (✪ depending on choice of flour mix)

225 g/8 oz flour mix (see page 158)
1/2 tsp salt
2 tsp wheat-free baking powder (see page 159)
30 g/1 oz dairy-free margarine
30 g/1 oz caster sugar
60 g/2 oz sultanas
soya milk to mix, approx 5 tbsp
1/2 tsp vanilla essence

Sift the flour into a bowl and add the salt and baking powder. Add the margarine and rub into a breadcrumb consistency. Stir in the sugar and sultanas. Stir the vanilla essence into the milk. Add the milk to mix into a soft but not sticky dough.

Roll out on a floured board and cut into 4 cm/1½ in rounds, brush the tops with milk and bake in the oven for 10–12 minutes at 200°C/400°F/Gas Mark 6.

Shortbread   ◆W◆M◆E

Makes 15–20 pieces (◆ depending on choice of flour mix)

225 g/8 oz flour mix (see page 158)
115 g/4 oz ground rice
115 g/4 oz caster sugar
225 g/8 oz dairy-free margarine
few drops pure almond essence (optional)

Mix together the flour, rice and sugar. Melt the fat in a saucepan and add the almond essence if using. Add to the dry ingredients and mix together well.

Roll out to 1 cm/1/2 in thickness, cut into shapes and pinch the edges.

Place on a baking sheet and bake at 180°C/350°F/Gas Mark 4 for about 30 minutes or until lightly golden. Leave to cool on a tray.

Honeyed ginger flapjacks   ◆W◆M◆E

Makes 8–10 fingers

225 g/8 oz millet flakes or rice flakes
140 g/5 oz sunflower oil (preferably 'buttery' variety)
85 g/3 oz light soft brown sugar
2 tbsp clear Mexican honey
1/3–1/2 tsp ground ginger (to taste)

Preheat the oven to 180°C/350°F/Gas Mark 4.

Pour the oil into a saucepan over a low heat and stir in the sugar, honey, flakes and ginger. Mix very thoroughly. Grease an 18 cm/7 in square shallow baking tin and press in the mixture.

Bake for 20–25 minutes until golden and lightly firm.

Mark into fingers while still hot. Leave in the tin until cold.

Granny's gingerbreads

Makes 8 approx   (depending on choice of flour mix)

115 g/4 oz dairy-free margarine
115 g/4 oz caster sugar
115 g/4 oz flour mix (see page 158)
1 tsp wheat-free baking powder (see page 159)
2 tsp ground ginger

Cream the margarine and sugar together until pale. Mix together the flour, baking powder and ginger. Add 1 tbsp of flour mix at a time to the cream mixture to form a stiff dough.

Roll into balls the size of a very small egg and place on a baking sheet, well apart.

Bake on the bottom shelf for 15 minutes at 180°C/ 350°F/Gas Mark 4. Then leave to cool on a wire tray.

Shortcrust pastry

To cover 20 cm/8 inch pie dish

170 g/6 oz flour mix (see page 158)
1/4 tsp salt
60 g/2 oz dairy-free margarine
30 g/1 oz white hard vegetable oil
1 egg, beaten, plus 1 tbsp water

Sift the flour into a bowl and add the salt. Add the fats and rub into a breadcrumb consistency. Add sufficient egg mixture to give a soft, but not sticky, dough.

Roll out on a floured board and use as required. If baking blind, bake at a slightly lower temperature than normal pastry, at about 180°C/350°F/Gas Mark 4.

Special occasion pastry

To cover 20 cm/8 inch pie dish

225 g/8 oz flour mix (see page 158)
1/4 tsp salt
60 g/2 oz dairy-free margarine
60 g/2 oz hard white vegetable oil
60 g/2 oz icing sugar
1 large egg, beaten
1/2 tsp pure almond essence

Sift the flour and salt into a bowl. Add the fats and rub into a fine breadcrumb consistency. Stir in the sugar.

Stir the almond essence into the beaten egg and add sufficient to the crumbs to combine and give a soft, but not sticky, dough. Wrap in film and chill for 20 minutes.

Roll out on a floured board and use as required. If baking blind, bake on a slightly lower temperature than normal pastry, at about 180°C/350°F/Gas Mark 4.

Rice cakes

Makes 8–10 cakes

170 g/6 oz flour mix (see page 158)
115 g/4 oz ground rice
1 1/2 tsp wheat-free baking powder (see page 159)
170 g/6 oz dairy-free margarine
170 g/6 oz caster sugar
3 eggs, beaten
pure almond essence
115 g/4 oz sultanas

Sift the flour, ground rice and baking powder together. Cream the margarine and sugar together, add the beaten eggs and almond essence a little at a time and gradually add the flour mix. Fold in the sultanas. If the mixture is too stiff, a little soya milk can be added.

Spoon into greased patty tins and bake at 190°C/375°F/Gas Mark 5 for 20 minutes.

If desired, a little water icing (120 g/4 oz icing sugar mixed with 3 tbsp warm water) can be spread over the centre of the cakes when cool.

Apple cake

For a 20 cm/8 inch cake tin

115 g/4 oz dairy-free margarine
115 g/4 oz caster sugar
few drops vanilla essence
2 large eggs, beaten
170 g/6 oz flour mix (see page 158)
1½ tsp wheat-free baking powder (see page 159)
225–280 g/8–10 oz cooking apples, peeled, cored and sliced

Topping
115 g/4 oz flour mix (see page 158)
85 g/3 oz dairy-free margarine
85 g/3 oz soft brown sugar
2 level tsp cinnamon

Cream the fat and sugar until pale and fluffy, add the vanilla essence to the eggs and add a little at a time to the creamed mixture. Fold in the flour mixed with the baking powder. Mix to a fairly stiff dropping consistency, if necessary adding a little hot water.

Turn into a lined 20 cm/8 in loose-bottomed cake tin. Arrange the sliced apples on top of the cake mixture.

To make the topping, rub the margarine into the flour and stir in the sugar and cinnamon. Spread the topping over the apples.

Bake at 180°C/350°F/Gas Mark 4 for 1–1¼ hours or until lightly golden brown. Leave in the tin to cool.

Iced almond cakes

Makes 12–16 cakes

225 g/8 oz ground rice
170 g/6 oz caster sugar
3 eggs
pure almond essence (to taste)
120 g/4 oz icing sugar
glacé cherries
3 tbsp warm water

Grease some very small cake tins. Whisk the sugar and the eggs together for 15 minutes. Add the almond essence and ground rice. Mix well together and pour into the prepared tins.

Bake at 190°C/375°F/Gas Mark 5 for 15–20 minutes. Remove from the oven, leave to stand for 5–10 minutes and place on a wire tray.

Coat the cakes with icing made from icing sugar and water and put half a glacé cherry on top of each cake. Serve in paper cases.

Coconut fruit tarts

Makes 12–16 tarts

225 g/8 oz wheat-free shortcrust pastry (see page 165)
apricot jam
1 egg
85 g/3 oz caster sugar or fructose
115 g/4 oz desiccated coconut
dried, ready-to-eat pineapple cubes

Preheat the oven to 190°C/375°F/Gas Mark 5.

Line greased patty tins with pastry and put ½ teaspoon jam in the base of each tart. In a basin, whisk the egg well, add the sugar and mix. Add the coconut and fold in until well mixed.

Put a heaped teaspoonful of the mixture into each tart and a pineapple cube in the centre.

Bake for 20 minutes or until golden brown.

Spiced fruity rock cakes

Makes 8–10 cakes

170 g/6 oz high-fibre flour mix (see page 158)
1¹/₂ tsp wheat-free baking powder (see page 159)
¹/₂ tsp mixed spice
pinch nutmeg
pinch cinnamon
85 g/3 oz dairy-free margarine
85 g/3 oz raisins
1¹/₂ oz glacé cherries, cut into pieces
1¹/₂ oz stem ginger, chopped
1 large egg, beaten
1–2 tbsp soya milk

Line a twelve-compartment patty tin with cake papers.

Sift the flour and spices into a bowl, add the margarine and rub into a breadcrumb consistency. Add the raisins, cherries and ginger. Stir to mix evenly.

Add the egg and enough milk to give a fairly stiff consistency. Divide the mixture between the paper cases.

Bake at 200°C/400°F/Gas Mark 5 for 15–20 minutes, or until cooked and lightly golden.

Chocolate cherry brownies

Makes approx 16 squares

85 g/3 oz carob dairy-free confectionery
60 g/2 oz dairy-free margarine
¹/₃ tsp pure vanilla essence
170 g/6 oz caster sugar
2 large eggs
85 g/3 oz flour mix plus 1 tsp wheat-free baking powder,
sifted together (see page 158)
40 g/1¹/₂ oz glacé cherries, washed, dried and cut into
pieces

Grease a 20 cm/8 in shallow square cake tin and line with baking parchment.

Melt the carob bar pieces in a bowl over a pan of hot water. Stir in the margarine until melted. Remove from the heat. Beat in the sugar and eggs mixed with the vanilla essence. Fold in the flour, dust the cherry pieces in flour and fold into the mixture.

Bake at 180°C/350°F/Gas Mark 4 for 25–30 minutes or until risen and firm to touch. Cut into squares.

Grandma's rice and apricot cake

For a 18 cm/7 inch cake tin

225 g/8 oz dairy-free margarine
225 g/8 oz caster sugar
170 g/6 oz flour mix with 2 tsp wheat-free baking powder
    added (see page 158)
115 g/4 oz ground rice
4 eggs
1/2 tsp almond essence (if not allowed, use vanilla)
tinned apricots in natural juice
little demerara sugar

Drain the juice from the apricots, dry and leave to one side. Grease and line a 18 cm/7 in cake tin.

Cream the margarine and sugar until pale, light and very fluffy. Mix the flour, baking powder and ground rice together. Add gradually in small amounts to the creamed margarine, alternating with beaten egg. Add the almond essence and beat to a smooth consistency. Pour into the cake tin.

Slice the apricots into thin slices, lay gently over the top of the mixture, sprinkle over the demerara sugar and bake at 150°C/325°F/Gas Mark 3. Test after an hour to see if the cake is cooked; it will take 1–1¼ hours.

Banana sultana cake

Makes 1 x 450 g/1 lb loaf

115 g/4 oz dairy-free margarine
60 g/2 oz caster sugar
2 large eggs
115 g/4 oz high-fibre flour mix and 1 tsp wheat-free baking
   powder, mixed together (see page 158)
2 ripe bananas, mashed
60 g/2 oz walnuts, pieces or chopped (optional)
60 g/2 oz sultanas
2–3 drops vanilla essence

Line a 450 g/1 lb loaf tin with baking parchment. Cream the
fat and sugar together until light and fluffy. Beat the eggs
together, adding the vanilla essence.

Beat in the eggs, half at a time, adding 1 tbsp of the flour
mix with the egg. Fold in the remaining flour mix and add the
bananas, sultanas and walnuts. Fold in until evenly mixed.

Bake in a preheated oven at 180°C/350°F/Gas Mark 4 for
45–55 minutes or until light and springy to touch.

This cake keeps for up to three days and is suitable for
freezing, whole or in individually wrapped slices.

Prune and apricot teabread

Makes 1 x 450 g/1 lb loaf

225 g/8 oz high-fibre flour mix plus 2 tsp wheat-free baking
   powder (see page 158)
1/2 tsp mixed spice
1/2 tsp cinnamon
pinch nutmeg
140 g/5 oz dairy-free margarine
140 g/5 oz dried ready-to-eat apricots, chopped
140 g/5 oz ready-to-eat prunes, chopped
60 g/2 oz soft brown sugar
3 eggs, beaten
little soya milk (if necessary)

Place the flour, baking powder and spices in a bowl and mix. Add the margarine and rub into a breadcrumb consistency.

Stir in the sugar, apricots and prunes, add the eggs a little at a time and mix to a soft dropping consistency. Add a little soya milk if needed.

Turn into a lightly greased and lined 450 g/1 lb in loaf tin and bake for about an hour at 180°C/350°F/Gas Mark 4, or until cooked.

Pineapple and ginger cake

Makes 1 x 900 g/2 lb loaf

225 g/8 oz high-fibre flour mix (see page 158)
2 tsp wheat-free baking powder (see page 159)
1 level tsp mixed spice
60 g/2 oz soft brown sugar
115 g/4 oz dairy-free margarine
3 eggs, beaten
3–4 tbsp pineapple and ginger jam
85 g/3 oz sultanas

Beat the flour, baking powder, spice, sugar, margarine and eggs together until well mixed. Stir in the jam. Dust the sultanas with a little extra flour mix and fold them into the mixture.

Put the cake mixture in a greased and lined 900 g/2 lb loaf tin. Bake for 1–1¼ hours at 160°C/325°F/Gas Mark 3. If the cake starts to crack, reduce the oven temperature to 145°C/ 300°F/Gas Mark 2. Cover the top of the cake with grease-proof paper if it is browning too much.

Coconut pyramids

Makes 8–10

225 g/8 oz desiccated coconut
115 g/4 oz caster sugar
1 large egg, well beaten

1/2 tsp vanilla essence
little red pure food colouring (cochineal)
little cold water

Mix the coconut with the sugar, then add the beaten egg and
vanilla essence and mix. If necessary, add a little cold water to
make the mixture stick together. Colour with cochineal to a
pale pink shade.

Take a mould or an egg-cup (rinsed well with cold water)
and fill with the coconut mixture, pressing down well. Shake
out the pyramids onto a greased baking sheet. Place in the
refrigerator to chill for a few hours.

Remove and bake at 180°C/350°F/Gas Mark 4 for 15–20
minutes.

Victoria sponge cake

For 2 x 15–18 cm/6–7 inch sandwich tins

170 g/6 oz flour mix plus 1 tsp wheat-free baking powder
    (see page 158)
170 g/6 oz dairy-free margarine
85 g/3 oz caster sugar
3 eggs, beaten, with few drops vanilla essence
1 tbsp hot water

Heat the oven to 190°C/375°F/Gas Mark 4. Grease and line
two 15–18 cm/6–7 in sandwich tins.

Cream the margarine and sugar until pale and fluffy. Add
a little egg and 1 dessertspoon of flour. Beat into the mixture
and continue adding egg a little at a time, beating well.

Fold in the flour sifted with the baking powder. Add water
and mix.

Divide the mixture between the two tins and bake for
20–25 minutes, or until lightly golden and firm to touch.
When cold, sandwich with jam or dairy-free buttercream
filling (see recipe on page 175).

Treacle scones

Makes 6–8 scones

225 g/8 oz flour mix (see page 158)
1/4 tsp salt
2 tsp wheat-free baking powder (see page 159)
1 tsp mixed spice
60 g/2 oz dairy-free margarine
60 g/2 oz caster sugar
1 egg, beaten
1 tbsp black treacle
2 tbsp soya milk (if necessary)

Sift the flour into a bowl and add the salt, baking powder and mixed spice. Mix together.

Add the margarine and rub into a breadcrumb consistency. Mix in the sugar. Add the treacle to the beaten egg and mix well to combine. Pour into the flour and mix into a soft, but not sticky, dough, adding a little soya milk if necessary.

Roll out the dough on a floured board and cut into 4 cm/ 1 1/2 in scones.

Bake in the oven at 200°C/400°F/Gas Mark 6 for 10–12 minutes, or until cooked.

Cinnamon shortbread

Makes 8–10 pieces

115 g/4 oz flour mix plus 1 tsp wheat-free baking powder
   (see page 158)
85 g/3 oz dairy-free margarine
115 g/4 oz caster sugar
2 egg yolks
2 level tsp cinnamon
little demerara sugar and cinnamon

Rub the margarine into the flour to a breadcrumb consistency. Stir in the sugar and cinnamon and add the egg yolks. It should be a fairly stiff dough. If necessary, add a little soya milk.

Roll out on a floured board to thickness of about 1 cm/ ½ in. Brush the top with soya milk and sprinkle with a mixture of demerara sugar and cinnamon.

Bake at 180°C/350°F/Gas Mark 4 for 15–20 minutes, or until lightly golden.

Pear and carob cake

115 g/4 oz dairy-free margarine
140 g/5 oz rice flour
30 g/1 oz carob flour
85 g/3 oz soya flour
115 g/4 oz brown sugar
2 pears, stewed, cooled and liquidized
1–2 tbsp soya milk
1 level tsp sodium bicarbonate in 2 tsp water
Filling:
60 g/2 oz dairy-free margarine
85 g/3 oz icing sugar

Preheat the oven to 180°C/350°F/Gas Mark 4.

Rub the margarine into the flours, then add the sugar. Mix thoroughly. Make a well in the centre and slowly stir in the pears and milk substitute until all the flour has been taken up; the mixture should be slightly sloppy. Add the bicarbonate of soda and water. Beat the mixture hard until it becomes smooth and fluffy. This is important: if the beating does not reach this stage the cake will be flat and unpalatable.

Turn immediately into two 18 cm/7 in greased cake tins. Bake for 25–30 minutes.

For the filling, cream the margarine, add sugar gradually and beat together.

When the cake is cool, sandwich the two halves together with the filling.

Rice Krispie cakes

Makes 20–24 cakes

2 tbsp honey or golden syrup
30 g/1 oz brown sugar
at least 30 g/1oz Rice Krispies

Heat the honey and sugar until the sugar dissolves. Stir in enough Rice Krispies to absorb the honey. Spoon into paper cases and leave to cool and harden.

Alternatives: chopped dates or 2 tsp carob flour may be added.

Iced gingernuts

Makes 12–16

30 g/1 oz dairy-free margarine
30 g/1 oz soft brown sugar
60 g/2 oz golden syrup
60 g/2 oz soya flour
30 g/1 oz rice flour
1 tsp wheat-free baking powder (see page 159)
1/2 tsp cream of tartar
1/2 tsp ground ginger
120 g/4 oz icing sugar
3 tbsp warm water

Preheat the oven to 180°C/350°F/Gas Mark 4.

Melt the margarine in a pan on low heat and stir in the golden syrup and sugar. Sift together the dry ingredients and then re-sift them into the pan. Stir to a firm paste. Take small spoonfuls and roll in the hands until smooth (walnut size), then flatten on a greased baking tray. Bake for 15–17 minutes.

Leave to cool, then mix together the sugar and water to make the water icing and decorate.

Date and millet squares

Makes 16 squares

225 g/8 oz dates, chopped
115 ml/4 fl oz apple juice
115 g/4 oz dairy-free margarine
170 g/6 oz soft brown sugar
115 g/4 oz rice or millet flour
170 g/6 oz millet flakes

Preheat the oven to 180°C/350°F/Gas Mark 4.

Put the dates in a pan, pour in the apple juice and cook over a gentle heat until the mixture is soft and pulpy (about 5 minutes). Chop the margarine into small pieces. Place the sugar, rice or millet flour and millet flakes in a bowl, add the chopped margarine and mix until all the ingredients are combined.

Grease a 18 x 23 cm/7 x 9 in baking tin. Divide the millet mixture in half. Press half the mixture firmly into the bottom of the tin and spread the date mixture over the top. Cover with the remaining millet mixture and press down firmly.

Bake for 35–40 minutes. Allow to cool in the tin. Cut into squares when cold.

Eggless fruit cake

For a 20 cm/8 in diameter cake tin

450 ml/3/4 pint water
115 g /4 oz currants
115 g/4 oz raisins
225 g/8 oz dairy-free margarine
170 g/6 oz demerara sugar
115 g/4 oz millet flour
115 g/4 oz rice flour
1 tbsp wheat-free baking powder (see page 159)
1 tsp bicarbonate of soda
1 tsp mixed spice

Preheat the oven to 190°C/375°F/Gas Mark 5.

Put the water, currants, raisins, margarine and sugar in a pan and bring to the boil. Simmer for 5 minutes. Leave to cool.

Sift the millet flour, rice flour, baking powder, bicarbonate of soda and mixed spice together three times. When the ingredients in the pan are quite cold mix them with the flour mixture until thoroughly combined.

Grease a loose-bottomed 20 cm/8 in cake tin with margarine. Fill with the mixture and bake for 2 hours. Leave the cake to cool in the tin for a few minutes before turning it onto a wire tray.

BEVERAGES

Honey cold-soother

honey
1 clove
1/4 tsp cinnamon
few grains nutmeg

Pour a mug of water into a pan, add a large spoonful of honey, the clove, cinnamon and nutmeg and bring to the boil, stirring continuously. Strain and cool for at least a few minutes before drinking.

Peppermint bracer

1–2 drops pure peppermint oil (use very sparingly)
few grains caster sugar
1–2 tbsp apple juice

Put the peppermint oil and sugar into a jug and pour on a mugful of hot water just off the boil. Stir in the apple juice. Leave to cool to a drinkable heat.

Mango and ginger warmer

1/2 mango, liquidized
300 ml/1/2 pint soya milk
pinch ground ginger
little honey if required

Gently heat the soya milk and stir in the ginger. When the milk is at the required heat, briskly stir in the liquidized mango.

Spicy cinnamon

300 ml/1/2 pint soya milk
generous pinch cinnamon
small pinch nutmeg
1 tbsp black treacle

Pour the milk into a saucepan, add the cinnamon, a few grains of nutmeg and the black treacle. Heat gently to just below boiling, stirring continuously.

Banana milkshake

1 ripe banana, cut into slices
1 mug or cup soya milk or rice milk, chilled
1/4 tsp soya yoghurt

Place all the ingredients in a liquidizer, process and chill.

Other fruit milkshakes

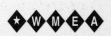

Take 3/4 tumbler of chilled soya milk or rice milk, some crushed ice and make your choice of milkshake by adding one of the following:

(a) 150 ml/1/4 pint raspberry purée
(b) few fresh strawberries

(c) few slices pineapple
(d) heaped tbsp blackcurrants
(e) rosehip syrup – follow instructions on bottle

Put the milk and fruit in a liquidizer, process until smooth, pour into a jug and add the crushed ice.

Fruit purée ◆WME A

If you prefer not to use milk, you can blend or liquidize the
    following:
1 pear, peeled, cored and chopped
2 or 3 apricots, depending on size, with crushed ice

Alternatively, try the 100 per cent pure green/white grape juice, now available from supermarkets, chilled with crushed ice and a drop of peppermint.

Vegetable drinks ◆WME

Most of us have our own favourite tomato juice recipes. Try adding carrot juice to yours with a pinch of salt. Possible new favourites include celery and cucumber with crushed ice.

Appendix

Foods containing cow's milk and cow's milk products

Milk is used in a variety of manufactured products. Check all labels on bought foods and if the following items are included do not use that product: milk, butter, margarine, cream, cheese, yoghurt, skimmed milk powder, non-fat milk solids, caseinates, whey, lactalbumin, lactose.

The foods listed below are likely to contain milk and/or milk products, so always check the list of ingredients.

biscuits
bread, bread mixes
breakfast cereals
cakes, cake mixes
gravy mixes
malted milk drinks, e.g. Horlicks, Ovaltine, Bournvita
puddings and mixes, e.g. ice-cream, instant whips,
    custards
ready meals – fish, meat, rice and pasta dishes
sauces, cream soups
sausages
sweets, e.g. milk chocolate, fudge, toffee
vegetables canned in sauce

Foods containing eggs

Foods containing egg yolk, egg white and lecithin should be avoided. The following may contain eggs:

> baked foods – cakes, biscuits, pastry and batter
> egg noodles and pasta
> lemon curd
> malted milk drinks, e.g. Bournvita
> mayonnaise
> puddings and mixes
> soups

Foods containing wheat

Wheat is present in the products listed below. Check all labels on manufactured foods. If wheat, wheat starch, edible starch, modified starch, cereal filler, cereal binder or cereal protein appear in the ingredients do not use that product. Foods marked with an asterix may or may not contain wheat.

Beverages

> cocoa,* drinking chocolate,* coffee essence,* milk shake flavourings,* Horlicks, Ovaltine*

Biscuits

> homemade and bought

Bread

> including white, wholemeal, wholewheat, granary breads, rye bread,* slimming bread

Breakfast cereals

> e.g. Shredded Wheat, Puffed Wheat, All-Bran, Weetabix, Shreddies, muesli,* baby cereals*

Cakes
including homemade and bought cakes, cake mixes and scones

Dairy products and fats
cheese spreads,* processed cheese,* packet suet*

Fish
tinned,* fish paste,* fish cooked in batter, breadcrumbs or a sauce

Flours and cereals
ordinary wheat flours, bran, wheatgerm, semolina, pasta, noodles

Fruit
pie fillings*

Meat
tinned,* ready meals,* pies, sausage rolls, meat paste,* pâté,* sausages*

Pastry
homemade, bought, mixes and frozen

Puddings
packet puddings, dessert mixes,* ice-cream,* mousses,* custard powder*

Vegetables
tinned in sauces, e.g. baked beans,* tinned vegetable salad,* instant potato powder*

Miscellaneous
stuffings, savoury spreads,* mayonnaise,* curry powder,* mustard,* chutney,* mincemeat,* peanut butter,* lemon curd,* sweets and chocolates,* baking powder,* gravy browning,* stock cubes,* soy sauce,* pepper compounds, packet seasonings

Foods containing yeast

The following products can, and frequently do, contain yeast in one form or another:

bread – any kind of bread, except soda bread

bread sauce, bread pudding, stuffings made with bread-crumbs, breadcrumb coatings on, e.g. fish fingers, fish cakes, potato croquettes

buns made with yeast, e.g. teacakes, rolls, crumpets, doughnuts

cheese, buttermilk, soured cream, synthetic cream

cream crackers, Twiglets

fermented beverages, e.g. wine, beer, cider

fruit juice (home squeezed citrus fruits are yeast-free)

yeast extract, Bovril, most stock cubes and gravy browning, tinned and packet soups

grapes, sultanas, currants, plums, dates, prunes and products containing these, e.g. fruit cake, mincemeat, muesli, raisin bran

malted milk drinks, e.g. Ovaltine, Horlicks

meat products containing bread, e.g. sausages, meat loaf, beefburgers

overripe fruit

pizza

puddings made with bread, e.g. apple charlotte, summer pudding

vinegar and pickled foods, e.g. pickled onions, pickled beetroot, sauces containing vinegar, e.g. tomato ketchup, salad dressing, mayonnaise

vitamin products – most B vitamin products contain yeast

Foods containing corn

The products listed below can, and frequently do, contain corn in one form or another, as cornstarch, oil, syrup or cornmeal. Modified starch, edible starch, food starch, maize oil, glucose syrup, vegetable oil and dextrose may also be derived from corn. Always check the label on manufactured products. Products marked with an asterisk may or may not contain corn.

baking mixtures for cakes and biscuits*
baking powders*
bleached white flour
bottle sauces – many contain food starch or syrup*
cakes and biscuits*
canned foods, e.g. soups, puddings, baked beans*
cornflakes
cornflour
custard powder
gravy browning
ices, ice-creams*
instant puddings*
instant teas, e.g. lemon tea mix contains dextrose
jams, jellies*
margarine and vegetable oils containing corn oil
peanut butter*
polenta
popcorn
salad dressings*
sweets – may be sweetened with corn syrup, e.g. sherbets, marshmallows
tortillas

Useful Addresses

Associations

British Migraine Association
178A High Road
Byfleet
West Byfleet
KT14 7ED

National Eczema Society
163 Eversholt Street
London
NW1 1BU
Tel: 0171 388 4097

The Coeliac Society
PO Box 220
High Wycombe
HP11 2HY

National Association for
Colitis and Crohn's Disease
98A London Road
St Albans
AL1 1NX
Tel: 01727 844296

The Arthritis Research
Campaign
Copeman House
St Mary's Court
St Mary's Gate
Chesterfield
S41 7TD

Supermarket Nutrition Services

These services provide
information on their
products, i.e. milk-free,
gluten-free etc.

Asda
Sue Malcolm, Dietician
Customer Services Dept
Asda Stores Ltd
South Bank
Great Wilson Street
Leeds
LS11 5AD
Tel: 0113 241 7730

Tesco
Customer Services
Tesco
Freepost
Baird Avenue
Dundee
DD1 9NF
Tel: 0800 50555

Sainsbury
Customer Services
J Sainsbury plc
Stamford House
Stamford Street
London
SE1 9LL
Tel: 0171 695 6000

Co-op
Customer Services
CWS Ltd
Freepost
MR9 473
Manchester
M4 8BA
Tel: 0800 317827

Waitrose
Nutrition Advice Service
Waitrose
Doncastle Road
Bracknell
Berks
RG12 8AY
Tel: 01344 424680

Boots
Miss V. Pennington
Boots the Chemists
Healthcare Business Unit
D90 East Building
Nottingham
NG90 1BS
Tel: 0115 9495 227

Marks & Spencer
Customer Services
Room 101
Marks & Spencer
Michael House
47 Baker Street
London
W1A 1DN
Tel: 0171 268 1234

Safeway
Nutrition Advice Service
Safeway plc
6 Millington Road
Hayes
Middlesex
UB3 4AY
Tel: 0181 848 8744

Somerfield
Customer Relations
Somerfield Stores Ltd
Whitchurch Lane
Bristol
BS14 0TJ
Tel: 0117 935 9359

Gluten-free products

Cantassium Company
225–229 Putney Bridge Road
London
SW15 2PY
Tel: 0181 874 1130
(Brand name: Trufree)

Dr Schar
PO Box 126
Worcester
WR3 7BR
Tel: 01905 28833
(Brand name: Schar)

General Dietary Ltd
PO Box 38
Kingston-upon-Thames
KT2 7YP
Tel: 0181-336-2323
(Brand names: Ener-G,
Valpiform, Tinkyada)

Gluten-Free Foods Limited
Unit 10, Honeypot Business
Park, Parr Road
Stanmore
HA7 1NL
Tel: 0181 952 0052
(Brand names: Barkat,
Clara's Kitchen, Glutano,
Tritamyl)

Lifestyle Healthcare Limited
Centenary Business Park
Station Road
Henley-on-Thames
RG8 1DS
Tel: 01491 411767
(Brand name: Lifestyle
Healthcare)

Nutricia Dietary Products
Newmarket Avenue
White Horse Business Park
Trowbridge
BA14 0QX
Tel: 01225 771801
(Brand names: Glutafin,
Rite-Diet)

SHS International Ltd
100 Wavertree Boulevard
Wavertree Technology Park
Liverpool
L7 9PT
Tel: 0151 228 1992
(Brand name: Juvela)

Ultrapharm Limited
Centenary Business Park
Henley-on-Thames
RG9 2AW
Tel: 01491 578 016
(Brand names: Aproten,
Arnotts, Bi-Aglut, Polial,
Ultra)

Index